THE
LIVING WILL

Consent to treatment at the end of life

Report under the auspices of
Age Concern Institute of Gerontology
and
Centre of Medical Law and Ethics
King's College, London

Edward Arnold
A division of Hodder & Stoughton
LONDON   NEW YORK   MELBOURNE   AUCKLAND

© 1988 Age Concern England

First published in Great Britain 1988

British Library Cataloguing in Publication Data
The livingwill : consent to treatment at the
    end of life.
    1. Health services. Patients. Therapy.
    Consent of patients. Ethical aspects.
    2. Great Britain. Health services. Patients.
    Therapy. Consent of patients to therapy.
    Legal aspects
    I. Age concern Institute of Gerontology
    II. King's College, London, *Centre of
    Medical Law and Ethics*
    174'.2

    ISBN 0-340-49142-6

Photoset in Linotron Sabon 10½/12pt by
Northern Phototypesetting Co, Bolton, England
Printed and bound in Great Britain
for Edward Arnold, the educational academic and medical publishing
division of Hodder and Stoughton Limited, 41 Bedford Square, London
WC1B 3DQ by Biddles Limited, Guildford and King's Lynn

Contents

Members of the Working Party

Professor Ian Kennedy LL M (Chairman), Professor of Medical Law and Ethics, King's College London

Dr Gerry Bennett MB, MRCP, Consultant Physician in Geriatric Medicine, The London Hospital (Mile End)

Ms Sally Greengross BA(Hons), FRSH, The Director, Age Concern England

Mr Andrew Grubb MA, Tutor and Law Fellow, Fitzwilliam College, Cambridge

Mrs Jill Martin LL M, Reader in Law, King's College London

Dr George Robertson MB, MD, FFA, Consultant Anaesthetist, Aberdeen Royal Infirmary

Dr David Greaves MB, M.Litt. (Secretary), Director of Research, Centre of Medical Law and Ethics, King's College, London

Preface

A major part of the work of Age Concern England is to draw
attention to the potential of elderly people and their needs.
'Celebrating Age' was thus its year-long campaign designed to
assert a positive view of old age and elderly people, showing
how rich, happy and fulfilling later life can be. But Age Concern, which serves as the National Council on Ageing, is also
eager to promote discussions of some of the long-term issues
which are pressing more and more urgently upon society
because an increasing number of elderly people are in need of
care as their lives draw to a close.

For this reason Age Concern welcomed the opportunity of
joining with the Centre of Medical Law and Ethics at King's
College, London, in setting up a working party to study the
medical, ethical and legal questions which arise when elderly
people who are no longer able to make their wishes known are
kept alive for prolonged periods by medical treatment and care,
which they might have refused if they had still been competent.

The report raises issues which have probably not been considered before in such a comprehensive way. The working
party does not feel that the time has come to make specific
recommendations, let alone to suggest draft legislation, but it
has set forth in some detail the range of options that are
available. It is to be hoped that the issues raised will be widely
discussed, not only by members of the caring professions but
also by lawyers and legislators.

Age Concern England thanks Professor Ian Kennedy and his
colleagues for this valuable contribution to what it hopes will
be an ongoing debate in the years ahead.

David Say
(The Rt. Revd Dr David Say, KCVO, Chairman, Age Concern
England)

Foreword

The working party was set up as a joint venture between Age Concern England and the Centre of Medical Law and Ethics of King's College London. Individual members were invited to join because of their personal interest and expertise in different aspects of the project.

The issues involved have not been considered before in a comprehensive manner within the British context. This meant that a great deal of material had to be reviewed and digested by the working party before the shape of the report began to emerge, but it also made the task both challenging and stimulating. The working party was small and one of its features was the degree to which every member made a substantial contribution, both in discussion and in drafting sections of the report.

We would like to acknowledge the help given us by two American visitors who are specialists in this subject: Professor John Stanley from Lawrence University, Wisconsin, and Professor Larry Heintz from the University of Hawaii. We also held a consultation meeting at which we received comments from some thirty people with a particular knowledge and interest prior to finalising the report.

Finally our thanks are due to Mrs Sylvia Seeley, who typed and retyped the drafts of the report and prepared copies, with her customary good humour and cheerfulness.

1 Introduction: The Nature and Scale of the Problem

Background: Stating the issue

There are increasing numbers of incurably ill and incapacitated people, many of whom are elderly, who can be kept alive for prolonged periods by medical treatment and care, but who are incompetent to consent to or refuse such management. In recent years concern has been expressed that many of these people have received treatment which they would have refused if they had remained competent. This applies especially to new drugs and technologies and relates in particular to life-sustaining treatment. And, of course, it is a continuing, some would say growing, area of concern.

Two main reasons have been advanced to explain why this situation warrants concern and calls for remedies. The first is the desire to respect the liberty of individuals and to protect them from the indignity, suffering and pain to which continued treatment may lead. The second relates to the social and economic costs, both to individual patients and families, and to the state, in looking after and treating large numbers of elderly and incapacitated people. The assumption in the second instance is that, given the opportunity to make their wishes known, a significant proportion of these people would opt for less or a different regime of treatment than is usually given with a consequent saving of resources.

If the need to change existing practices is accepted, two potential routes may be considered, which should be seen as complementary rather than mutually exclusive. Firstly, doctors may be persuaded to make changes in their practice. Secondly, advance directives may be introduced either on a statutory or non-stautory basis. An advance directive is the generic term for an act whereby a person, whilst competent, specifically makes arrangements about his future health care decisions should he become incompetent. This may be achieved either by an instrument which has become known as a living will, or by a durable (or enduring) power of attorney (or a combination of both).

The term 'living will' refers to a document in which a person, while still competent, requests and directs that certain measures, which may be variously specified, should be adopted if and when he becomes incapable of taking responsibility for his own health care, i.e. by consenting to or refusing treatment. The measures usually relate to the refusal of certain forms of treatment aimed at the preservation of the person's life. A durable (or enduring) power of attorney in the context of health care, allows a person, whilst competent, to appoint an agent to act on his behalf, in specified matters of health care, if and when he becomes incompetent.

Clearly, the most formal method of establishing the principle of advance directives is by legislation. This was first mooted in the USA. In 1976 California became the first State to pass a 'Natural Death Act' which gave recognition to the principle of living wills.[1] Since then the majority of States in the USA have enacted legislation relating to living wills, durable powers of attorney, or a combination of the two. In the UK no such legislation has been enacted or contemplated. In its absence there is considerable uncertainty about the present legal position, as well as about what may be ethically proper. Furthermore, there is no clear picture of what exactly happens in current medical practice in relation to non-treatment decisions.

As regards what should be done, there is a wide range of views, and several different approaches can be identified:

(1) The concept of advance directives is morally wrong because in no circumstance has any person the right to refuse measures which will prolong life. This 'sanctity of life' view precludes any consideration of legislation to introduce living wills and clearly limits the range of options available to the doctor in his care of the patient.

(2) There is no need to introduce legislation concerning

advance directives because it is already legally and morally permissible to 'allow people to die' in certain circumstances and this is reflected in good medical practice. This view has been clearly voiced by the Law Reform Commission of Canada – 'The decision to terminate or not to initiate useless treatment is sound medical practice and should legally be recognised as such. The law, then, should not begin from the principle that a doctor who fails to prolong life acts illegally, but rather from the principle that a doctor acts legally if he does not prolong death'.[2] Whilst rejecting the need for advance directives, this view does indicate the need for clarification of the legal position so that it may reflect or establish good medical practice. In the UK the British Medical Association has also expressed its opposition to legislation. In defence of the status quo the Association argues that its decision 'does not affect the current situation, in that any patient may express his wishes, either orally or in writing, to his general practitioner, who will then be aware of the patient's wishes in this respect'.[3] This does not ensure that the patient's wishes will be respected though, because the general practitioner will only follow them if he sees fit. Furthermore, such mechanisms for the expression of particular wishes are not widely known to the general public.

(3) The position in law is confused and, as a consequence, practice varies.

Doctors are uncertain about the law relating to withholding or withdrawing treatment and this has led to arbitrariness in practice. This is an unsatisfactory situation which calls for prompt action. Two lines of approach may be proposed:

(a) that the time has come to introduce legislation concerning advance directives. Following the models already available in many States of the USA, this could involve living wills, durable powers of attorney or some combination of the two. In the UK, proposals have already been made in respect of living wills, and suggestions put forward on the form they might take – 'People should be encouraged to declare their own wishes in writing before reaching senility . . . A signed statement would have legal standing in the sense that it would be drafted within a legal framework to exclude the influence of any person who might have an interest in the early demise of the patient. However, it would not be legally binding upon any future decision – it would be a statement of wish which would not necessitate any reciprocal commitment'.[4]

(b) that the situation should be reviewed and analysed before suggesting proposals about how to improve it. Alternative strategies, both statutory and non-statutory, should be considered and their consequences carefully weighed before any final decisions are taken. The guiding principle should be respect for the autonomy of individuals and attention paid to how far different strategies might reflect this in practice. Other considerations, such as the possible social and economic consequences of any proposed change, must also be taken into account.

Neither of the two views (1) and (2) set out above is consistent with maximising respect for the liberty of individuals and autonomous decision-making. In each case it is the opinion of others which is to count in determining the care a patient receives. In the case of (1), an absolute 'sanctity of life' principle precludes any possibility of choice, let alone autonomous choice. In the case of (2), it is the doctors who decide, within a legal framework which, because of its uncertainty, may be interpreted restrictively or extremely permissively. It follows that what is done in practice tends to be conflated with what ought to be done.

Only (3) above turns away from these paternalistic stances and attempts to respect individual autonomy. To move immediately to a consideration of possible legislation aimed at giving expression to this principle would, however, allow no opportunity to consider and weigh the possible pitfalls and alternatives. The approach adopted in this report, therefore, will be to proceed more slowly. The aim is to examine the current state of the law and of medical practice and then make recommendations in the light of these.

Background: The medical context

In recent years there has been a growing public and professional interest in and concern about the treatment of the terminally ill and the elderly. Much of this concern has arisen from the increase in sophisticated medical technology which is available to doctors to maintain a patient's life where in the past nature would have taken its course and the patient would have died. The problem has been referred to repeatedly in the medical literature. For example:

. . . medicine has reached the point at which its capacity to maintain life or at any rate some vestigial form of life has outstripped its ability to assure the quality of that life.[5]

. . . our technological ability to manipulate the human body exponentially exceeds our moral capacity to decide on such manipulations.[6]

What the public, as distinct from doctors, may think is difficult to know. There are only a few surveys of public attitudes in relation to these issues. One conducted in 1983 by the American Hospital Association showed that about 75 per cent of the Americans surveyed thought doctors should discontinue life-support systems on patients for whom there is little or no hope of recovery and leading a normal life. Discontinuance was favoured by a higher proportion of elderly than young people.[7] Another American survey found that 71 per cent of people thought that life-support systems of hopelessly ill patients should be discontinued.[8] A further study of patients with varying degrees of heart or liver disease concluded that 75 per cent would want to refuse tube feeding or intensive care if they had severe senile dementia.[9] A British survey was carried out by MORI in 1984. In response to the question 'Suppose a person has a painful incurable disease, do you think that doctors should be allowed by law to end that patient's life if the patient requests it?', 75 per cent of the sample replied 'Yes', 24 per cent replied 'No'.[10] Although these surveys did not relate directly to the use of advance directives, they do indicate that a majority of the public, both in Britain and the USA, accept that there are times when it is appropriate to forego life-sustaining treatment (indeed the British survey goes further in suggesting widespread support for the view that the doctor be permitted to kill the patient, a view which does not form part of this report). A large section of the public believes that there are medical interventions which in some circumstances produce a result worse than death itself. These might include the use of life-support equipment for a patient in a persistent vegetative state, or subjecting a severely disabled patient to cardiopulmonary resuscitation, or artificial feeding in a patient with advanced senile dementia.

Some people amongst those groups being considered already fear that going into hospital may spell death, because a doctor might decide that a life is no longer worthwhile, and either withdraw treatment or actively bring about death as quickly as possible. Some doctors and patients might see in the notion of foregoing treatment at the request of a patient an implicit condonation or encouragement of suicide or homicide. Even if it was never actually practised there might still be fear and suspicion. It must be made clear, therefore, that such conduct would be unlawful and that nothing in this report is intended to lend support to such a position.

If the directive calls for some positive act of killing on the part of the doctor such an act would also be unlawful. Consequently, an advance directive which called for it would be invalid. To change the law would appear to be in keeping with the logic of respect for autonomy reflected in this report. But this is, perhaps, to give too much emphasis to the autonomy of the patient and ignore the autonomy of others, including the doctor, and the potential contingent risks which could flow from such a step. It remains ultimately for Parliament whether the law should be changed in this regard, and will not be considered further as it is beyond the remit of this report.

Conclusion

There is a wide range of medical conditions which may lead to permanent disability and incompetence. In these circumstances the unquestioned application of all possible medical treatment and care may not be desired by a majority of the public and is morally debatable. As regards the law, many of those who are involved feel that the situation is unclear, leaving both doctor and patient in a position of uncertainty. The suggestion is that this may give rise to unacceptable variability in medical practice.

It is these questions that are examined in this report, covering the medical, ethical and legal issues involved. A set of practical proposals have been developed based on these findings, detailing how best to improve the situation.

References

1. California Health and Safety Code – The Natural Death Act. Sections 7185–95 (West Supplement, 1978).
2. Law Reform Commission of Canada (1982). *Euthanasia, Aiding Suicide and Cessation of Treatment.* Working Paper 28, p. 69.
3. Letter from the British Medical Association to Age Concern England (1984).
4. Robertson, G. S. (1982). Dealing with the brain-damaged old: Dignity before sanctity. *Journal of Medical Ethics,* 8: 173–179.
5. Tindall, G. (1986). High-tech medicine: When to say no. *Journal of the Royal Society of Medicine,* 79: 56–7.
6. Emson, H. E. (1983). Rationing health care: Where does the buck stop? *Canadian Medical Association Journal,* 128: 435–8.
7. The Society for the Right to Die (1984). *Handbook of Living Will Laws, 1981–1984,* p. 7. The Society for the Right to Die, New York.
8. Dunea, G. (1983) When to stop treatment. *British Medical Journal,* 287: 1056–7.
9. Lo, B., McLeod, G. A. and Saika, G. (1986). Patient attitudes to discussing life–sustaining treatment. *Archives of Internal Medicine,* 146: 1613–15.
10. Jowell, R., Witherspoon, S. and Brock, L. (Eds) (1986). *British Social Attitudes: the 1986 Report,* p. 159. Gower, Aldershot.

2 Good Medical Practice

Introduction

Much of the debate concerning the care of the hopelessly ill patient, as has been seen in Chapter 1, begins with a double uncertainty. Firstly, what can modern medicine do for the patient; what techniques are available to comfort and ease the patient's suffering? Secondly, what does the law allow the doctor to do, and of what significance is it that a patient has expressed the wish to die with dignity?

In this chapter we are concerned with responding to the first of these two questions, and the subsequent chapter will deal similarly with the second relating to the existing law.

The analysis of these two issues is clearly a necessary precursor to any consideration of the need for changes in the law. For, if it appears that current law and available medical techniques do in fact meet the needs of those with whom we are concerned, then no changes are called for. All that is required is better understanding and awareness by doctors and patients.

We focus particularly on three groups of patients – the terminally ill, those who are seriously and permanently ill or disabled and who are not terminally ill but who would die if not treated, and those with irreversible dementia who are not dying but who require long-term 24-hour care. Although we are principally concerned with those who are incompetent, we shall also consider the care of those who are competent. We do so because it is important to identify what choices the law allows to the competent. These, we submit, should be considered as the background against which the law relating to the treatment of those no longer capable of making their own choices should be examined.

The structure of the chapter is as follows. Firstly, we attempt to provide working definitions of the three groups of patients discussed above. Secondly, we examine the treatment available to the three groups of patients, and the medical and social factors relevant to good medical practice in this area.

Definitions

As regards the three groups of patients identified above, it is important to understand at the outset those to whom this report applies. The first group is the terminally ill. A terminally ill patient is one who as a result of some illness, injury or degeneration of his mental or physical faculties will die within a relatively short and approximately quantifiable period of time, and for whom there is no prospect of long-term recovery even with medical intervention.

It will be obvious that the definition contains imprecise terms. It must necessarily do so. It is a matter of degree and opinion whether one regards a patient whose illness will kill him in one year as opposed to three months as terminally ill, and documents which state a specific time period range between these limits. Nevertheless, we feel that the definition given is sufficient for our purpose.

It will be clear from this definition that the irreversibly comatose individual is not to be regarded as terminally ill. Instead, we consider that such a person would fall within our second group of patients who require treatment to remain alive but who may survive for years if this is carried out. Others who would fall within this category would be patients requiring life-support to maintain survival but who suffer from no other underlying physical defect which would prove fatal, for example, a patient with permanent brain damage caused by drug overdosage.

The third category of patients are those suffering from irreversible dementia but who have no other illness which affects their mental capacity. Their treatment must relate to matters of hygiene, feeding and medication to control the symptoms of their mental illness. Many, but by no means all of these patients, could be detained under the provisions of the Mental Health Act 1983 and the legality of their treatment would be dictated by the terms of that Act.

Good medical practice

In the care of the terminally ill, those who are seriously and permanently ill or disabled, and those with dementia of severe degree, it is important to ask and attempt to define what constitutes good medical practice. Most of these people are elderly. There are no clearly defined guidelines apart from what is permissible by law and many people are unhappy at certain aspects of the care of these groups in both institutional and community settings. Any understanding of what is good medical practice must start with a full appreciation of the client group involved and of the individual features and circumstances of each particular patient.

Fundamental to the evaluation of each case is the time-honoured system of medical history taking and full physical examination. In the context of the groups under discussion, there is an additional need to assess formal and informal care networks together with psychological and social needs. It is becoming increasingly recognised that, within domestic and community settings, it is also vital to recognise the needs of carers.

By adopting this whole person approach, involving assessment by several disciplines, it is possible to form a picture, albeit at times an inadequate one, of an individual's life and circumstances as they relate to his medical condition. In hospital the greatest contribution to this process is usually made by nurses, using nursing records as part of problem-orientated care. (These records often present verbatim transcripts of patients' statements and wishes.)

In the care of long-stay and terminal patients, nurses have more frequent, prolonged and personal contact with patients and relatives than have the medical team, and so the opinions of nursing staff are vitally important in assessing the medical and ethical problems of patient management. In the past, nurses' views have not been given appropriate recognition.[1] The medical management of a clinical dilemma which involves ethical considerations should be decided by a process of open communication between the patient, doctors, nurses, relatives and other carers, and important conclusions should be recorded in the case notes.

The notion of 'quality of life' is essential in this process of assessment and decision-making. It is an elusive concept, but various attempts have been made to define it. It has been suggested that, for the individual, quality of life '. . . is a result of his/her consumption of market goods/leisure, public goods and other characteristics (physical and social) of the environment in which he/she is located'.[2] In the context of the frail elderly, however, Denham feels that measures of quality of life must include health (mortality and survival), health perception, function and mental health. He also stresses the importance of feeling (life satisfaction), life domain and the importance of the quality of the environment.[3] Attempts to define quality of life have also been made in relation to the elderly in the community.[4,5]

An 81-year-old American woman wrote with reference to her fellow ward patients, 'One can hardly call being fed, bathed, clothed and changed, and knowing nothing at all really living'.[6] The problem is to define what is meaningful living for the individual. Some argue that an evaluation of quality of life is impossible because the data are too 'soft', meaning that they are difficult to quantify and are not objective. Others argue that soft data can be made harder by using observations from a large number of studies in many different centres.

In the areas of intensive care, terminal malignant disease, cardio-pulmonary resuscitation and dementia, several attempts have been made to develop valid systems for quantifying jointly the stage of a disease, its prognosis, and the burdens on the individual in such a way as to allow an objective evaluation of the quality of life. Well-designed studies have an important place in setting the standards of good medical practice in all these areas of care, although at present these indicators or scoring systems have achieved greater recognition and validity in, for example, intensive care than in dementia.

However, these objective evaluations cannot provide a basis for decision-making on their own. They can only supply the information to allow individuals to make their own personal quality of life judgments and consequent decisions on treatment or non-treatment. Thus, in decisions on what constitutes good practice for those with an advanced and irremediable illness, an appreciation of the patient's own weighing of the circumstances should be sought whenever possible. Pearlman puts it thus:

Responsible use of the inherently ambiguous concept of quality of life occurs when clinicians attune their interactions with patients to the values and goals of the patient.[8]

Terminal care (see Appendix: Case 1)

Hospices, despite their rapid growth, currently care for only about five per cent of all those dying each year.[9] However, in their teaching role they are exerting a far greater influence, by raising the standards of terminal care for those people dying in hospital or at home. They have demonstrated that the science of symptom relief and the art of nursing care are integral and well matched. Dying should occur without distressing symptoms and without distress to patients.

At present, health care professionals often deal badly with the dying. The reasons are numerous and complex: lack of awareness of the type and degree of pain and other symptoms; lack of knowledge concerning the best therapy for a specific symptom; poor awareness of the attitudes and wishes of both patients and relatives. A British study of a large random sample of non-sudden deaths in hospital and at home found that community nurses rated the quality of terminal life as poor in 44 per cent of cases. Uncontrolled pain was reported by relatives in 54 per cent of patients, and a high proportion of relatives complained of apparently pointless over-treatment.[10] Many of these deficiencies could be resolved by better communication between professionals and patients and their relatives, especially concerning the objectives in terminal care. There is also a need to devise and implement better, more rapid and more responsive means of transmitting information between the relevant professionals in both the hospital and the community.

(a) *Pain control*

Pain can be a significant problem in advanced cancer, but the majority of patients can be relieved of it without specialist intervention. There is often hesitation in providing adequate pain relief because of the fear of being seen to hasten the end of life. In terminal cancer, the goal must be full pain relief, no breakthrough pain (which may occur if drugs are given too infrequently), and as few unwanted side-effects as possible. Only in the later stages should drug dosage cause significant impairment of consciousness, and then the relief of pain is part of the dying process and not the cause of it. However, it is not simply a matter of analgesia (pain relief) – pain is a perception influenced by emotion, and so it can be altered by fear, weakness and tiredness – hence the broad approach needed. Patients often have more than one type of pain, and management involves attention to the details of each separate source of pain or discomfort. The art of nursing the terminally ill person involves communication, listening and responding to fears and anxieties. Prevention of other complications such as pressure sores is essential, and continence aids can make a patient comfortable and less exhausted.

(b) *The role of the primary care services*

There are many aspects of terminal care which require particular expertise and insight, and for patients dying at home the relationship between the patient's general practitioner (GP) and family may be much closer and more supportive than in a hospital setting. The GP often makes the initial diagnosis or is involved on discharge from hospital. Apart from having an understanding of the patient's physical problem, the GP will be able to understand the patient within the context of the whole family. Some relatives discourage a terminally ill or elderly family member from discussing death because it is regarded as morbid. However, there is much evidence that open and honest discussion in terminal illness may be of benefit to both patients and relatives.

To deal with the various situations which may arise, there should be a network of support which may involve all the primary health care services, the social services, as well as specialist services such as psychiatry (for the treatment of depression), bereavement counselling, home terminal care schemes, pain-relief clinics and in-patient hospice care. The role of the Practice Nurse or District Nurse may be critical, and such carers may be given considerable discretion to increase dosage of pain-killing drugs when necessary. Invaluable support may also be obtained from neighbours, friends, churches and self-help groups.

This brief summary has focused only on particular areas in the care of the terminally ill. It is intended to be a stimulus to further reading and understanding, and to illustrate that it is often ignorance that leads health care professionals to deal badly with the dying, thus serving to reinforce prejudice and fear in the lay public.

The seriously and permanently ill or disabled
(see Appendix: Case 2)

Numerous conditions result in a person becoming seriously or permanently ill or disabled. In younger age groups, congential handicaps and conditions such as multiple sclerosis and the *sequelae* of road traffic accidents predominate. In older people the most common seriously disabling condition is stroke, foll-owed by arthritis, Parkinson's disease, heart failure and ob-structive airways disease, and the combined effects of severe physical and mental frailty. Those in the younger age groups (under 65) who require long-term institutionalised care by virtue of disability are usually looked after in units for the 'young chronic sick'.

After the age of retirement, the only alternative to being nursed at home by family and community support used to be long-stay continuous care in an NHS hospital setting, unless personal wealth allowed the use of private facilities. Long-stay wards were where geriatric medicine was born, and the negative image which they projected was the stimulus to changing the face and standards of medicine for the elderly. Traditionally elderly permanently ill or disabled people have been nursed in large traditional wards with few nurses and even less in the way of paramedical support. The general quality of care was poor, but standards within this type of setting have gradually improved. Luminaries in the field, such as Professor Peter Millard, have been instrumental in improving the quality of care for the long-stay elderly by asking awkward questions of health authorities regarding the levels of financing for the care of these patients.[11,12]

Other countries provided more resources many years ago. For example, in Scandinavia, admission to a long-stay unit ensures the provision of an individual room and bathroom.[13,14] In the UK it is gradually being acknowledged that such amenities are a basic prerequisite of good long-stay care, allowing for personal space, dignity and independence despite grave handicaps.

Complementary to the need for improved facilities is the need for trained nursing staff with the dedication and specialised knowledge to meet the enhanced expectations of patients and the public. Centres of excellence attend to all the detailed needs of daily living, including the provision of therapy for maintenance rather than improvement, the prevention of medical complications, the supply of aids to help with physical handicap, and the availability of mental and spiritual support. Patient committees and relative support groups also enhance the autonomy of institutionalised residents.

In recent years there have been fundamental reviews of the various alternatives to long-stay hospital care of the elderly and severely handicapped. In some areas, the policy of encouraging the provision of private nursing home and residential home facilities by the use of DHSS Supplementary Benefit funding has revolutionised working practices.[15,16] Some hospital units for the elderly now have very few or no long-stay continuous care beds, with almost their entire chronic sick population being cared for in the private sector. This policy is a source of continuing controversy, but what remains true is that this group of people has some of the most pressing needs in terms of overall care, and it is essential to seek the optimal proportion of medical, nursing, paramedical and other caring staff.

Care in hospital beds is expensive, and it is increasingly accepted that they should be mainly reserved for acute and rehabilitative care rather than long-stay care. There is thus an important need for assessment procedures for those who may require long-stay care.[17] Many seriously and permanently ill or disabled elderly people will also have some element of mental deterioration, but this may be delayed or mitigated by techniques such as 'reality orientation'.[18] Small units can be seen as resource centres for the community as a whole, where the skills developed can be used in such settings as old people's homes, units for younger people (e.g. behaviour modification centres) and other institutions. However, in spite of optimal care in the most appropriate environment, many elderly patients will become progressively more disabled and will present a greater number of physical and mental problems.

Confusion and dementia *(see Appendix: Case 3)*

Ten per cent of those over the age of 65 and 20 per cent of those over 80 suffer from chronic confusional states due to some form of dementia.[19] Dementia in the elderly usually leads to a progressive deterioration in mental function, often with related emotional disturbance, due to a gradual and irreversible loss of brain cells. Although some ten per cent of cases are precipitated by a reversible cause, for the majority there is no medical treatment which can affect its course with certainty.[20] About 60 per cent of cases are due to senile dementia of the Alzheimer type (SDAT), and the remainder are either related to arterial disease causing damage to multiple small areas of the brain, or have features of both types of dementia.[21]

Good medical practice must begin with accurate diagnosis. Many elderly people present to a health care setting with acute confusion (i.e. with an onset of hours or days, and a duration of less than three months). However, confusion is not a diagnosis in itself but a symptom of an underlying disease, and if a precipitating illness can be identified and treated, the patient may be restored to his pre-existing state of mental function. If a confusional state develops suddenly or there is evidence of a head injury, special investigations such as CT (computerised tomography) brain scanning may be valuable in establishing the diagnosis.

A deterioration in mental function may be more insidious and lead to a chronic confusional state (i.e. duration of more than three months). Although reversible causes may still be detected, including depression, vitamin deficiencies or an underactive thyroid, the likely diagnosis will be one of the dementing disorders.

An early feature of dementia is loss of memory, and it is important to exclude alternative causes of memory loss. The recent development of 'memory clinics'[22] has not only allowed the differentiation of the various causes of memory loss (some of which are benign and reversible), but such clinics also act as centres of teaching and research.

Since the later stages of dementia always lead to mental incompetence with an inability to manage personal and social affairs, it is probably the most common condition in which some form of advance directive might be considered appropriate. By this means the individual would be able to retain some control over his life despite the onset of a mentally incapacitating disease. Much would depend, however, on the ability to define the stage and prognosis of the condition with some certainty. In the past few years there have been attempts at predicting the outcome of dementia.[23] One recent American study claims greatly enhanced precision in establishing the exact stage in the progression of dementia, and concludes that it is now possible 'to sketch the clinical course of Alzheimer's Disease (a form of senile dementia) in universal, readily discernible terms'.[24] Such precision would improve the quality of decision-making in establishing guidelines for good medical practice in the treatment of elderly patients with dementia.

Intensive care and resuscitation

With the development of realistic guidelines of good medical practice, it should be possible to encourage doctors to examine critically their criteria for deciding when to use intensive care facilities. Hitherto, this area of practice has been beset by dilemmas in which distress to patients and relatives, quality of life, cost and futility have had to be weighed in the balance. The difficulties have been compounded by a lack of firm scientific data to allow the clinical evaluation to be objective. A consequence has been a long history of arbitrariness or indecision in which non-medical commentators have become more and more resentful of what can seem to be over-zealous and misplaced endeavours.

In response to public and medical concern, there have been several important steps in providing a more objective and scientific foundation for decision-making involving intensive care and resuscitation. In 1980 the Glasgow Coma Scale was devised as a means of predicting at an early stage those patients with head injuries who were most unlikely to make a meaningful recovery and in whom intensive care would therefore be inappropriate.[25] In the broader field of intensive care involving other categories of very ill patients, several reliable systems have been devised for minimising the risk of over-treatment by defining those clinical categories where the outcome is uniformly poor.[26]

In 1986 the British Intensive Care Society decided to promote the use of 'APACHE' (Acute Physiological and Chronic Health Evaluation) scores which were developed several years ago in the USA.[27] APACHE scores are derived from the presence of a range of selected clinical observations and measurements. The background research for the APACHE score was based upon studies of 6000 intensive care patients, and so forms a reliable basis for determining the desirability of using intensive care facilities.

Ever since the development of external heart massage in 1960, it has been a straightforward process to begin cardiopulmonary resuscitation (CPR) and it has become routine in some centres. The widespread use of CPR has come to mean that the dying process may often be insensitively subjected to physical intrusion. By way of contrast, a survey of residents in a large American home for the elderly showed that only six per cent would opt for CPR if their heart stopped, and almost 50 per cent would not want CPR. The remainder would leave the doctor to decide at the time of such an event.[28] Recent studies in Britain and America in patients suffering a cardiac arrest have begun to pinpoint those circumstances where the prognosis is such that it might be inappropriate to carry out CPR.[29,30]

The current status of the ethics of resuscitation in Britain was reviewed recently in the British Medical Journal.[31] The author concluded: 'The need is clear for us to ensure that futile attempts at resuscitation are minimised and that the modern medical profession does not get a name for prolonging misery and the process of dying simply because we are afraid to make a decision'. Thus there is a gradual move against routine CPR in favour of its more selective use. It is inevitable that large numbers of uncertain cases will remain, and in a finely balanced situation the worst and most worrying outcome is that of the patient whose heart is successfully restarted but whose brain is permanently damaged.

Artificial feeding and hydration

One of the relatively frequent dilemmas in caring for gravely ill patients (whether with terminal cancer, advanced senile dementia or severe stroke) is whether or not to institute or continue the giving of nutrition and fluids by artificial means. There are those who believe, in good faith, that the human physical need for food and water is so fundamental that it constitutes one of the components of basic comfort-care. This would mean that all patients with advanced and incurable illness who became unable or unwilling to eat and drink should routinely be given artificial feeding. This could be by a naso-gastric tube or a gastrostomy in the stomach, or by intravenous (parenteral) means.

Parenteral feeding, in which a high intake of calories can be administered into the bloodstream, has now been developed into a valuable and safe procedure which can be maintained for prolonged periods. Its main use is in patients with non-malignant conditions of the intestine which may be temporary or long lasting. However, it is possible to extend the use of parenteral feeding nowadays to include those dying of a malignant or other condition in which life is threatened because of lack of nutrition. The maintenance of normal hydration by intravenous fluids is an even simpler clinical routine than parenteral feeding.

Whether or not to give intravenous fluid is clearly more of a moral than a medical problem, which has hitherto been addressed in terms of the now outmoded ethical concept of ordinary and extraordinary means as originally employed (see Chapter 3). The comatose, dying patient would be quite unaware of thirst or hunger, and many intravenous regimens do not provide adequate hydration anyway, but appear to be used only to retain venous access for no clearly defined reason.

It is now acknowledged that artificial feeding and hydration, like any other treatment for the hopelessly ill patient, should have a recognisable goal which is medically and ethically desirable. Any benefits need to be weighed carefully against the burdensome aspects for a particular patient: 'tube feedings may be painful, invasive and impersonal for some patients, and . . . tying patients down to allow tube feedings is difficult to reconcile with the goal of humane care'.[32]

Physical surroundings/personal care and dignity

Fear of growing old with mental frailty is usually accompanied by a 'mind's eye' image of slovenly and dirty clothes, uncontrolled incontinence, disruptive behaviour or a dulled 'twilight' life of drug-induced stupor in a Victorian workhouse setting. This image is uncomfortable because it has an unpleasantly realistic basis. What can and does happen where imagination and resources are combined is a very different picture.

The elderly mentally infirm can be supported at home in familiar surroundings given enough community support. This should not mean a home help only twice a week and an unending commitment on family or friends, but a well planned support network. Day care, day and night sitters, community psychiatric nurses, voluntary workers, family aids, GP support and the use of respite admissions can keep patient, family and dignity intact.

Institutional care is needed for some people. With well decorated single rooms, innovative use of reality orientation techniques, trained staff in sufficient resident-to-staff ratios and the use of personal effects, many of the horrors of institutional care can be lessened.[33] Everyone should be dressed appropriately, preferably in their own clothes including underwear.

Continence can be achieved in most and those who need aids can be kept dry and odour-free unobtrusively. Behaviour modifications can help aggressive tendencies, while medication should be kept to a minimum. Good architectural design allows for wandering without harm (e.g. racetrack design). Residents often improve behaviourally and physically when the above conditions apply. Underlying processes continue but rates of mental decline can be markedly lessened.

A sudden worsening of physical condition or behaviour which is not life-threatening often implies an intercurrent medical problem, i.e. acute on chronic disease. These aspects should be investigated and treated, not only to relieve unpleasant symptoms, but to stop preventable deterioration and a slipping by default into the very state that so many abhor.

Excellent physical care of the elderly mentally infirm goes some way to negating the fear of becoming 'demented'.

Conclusion

The above discussion of good medical practice as it relates to the terminally ill, seriously and permanently ill or disabled and those with severe dementia, sets out the foundation upon which care should be provided and by reference to which difficult ethical decisions should be made. For patients within each of these groups, there may come a time when both medically and ethically consideration should be given to withdrawing or withholding further treatment. The ethical and legal framework within which these complex decisions should be considered is set out in the next chapter.

References

1. Wilson-Barnett, J. (1986). Ethical dilemmas in nursing. *Journal of Medical Ethics*, 3: 123–6.
2. Gillingham, R. and Reece, W. S. (1979). A new approach to quality of life measurement. *Urban Studies*, 16(3): 329–32.
3. Denham, M. (1983). Assessment of quality of life. In *Care of the long stay elderly patient*, pp. 21–43. Croom Helm, Kent.
4. George, L. and Bearon, L. B. (1980). *Quality of life in older persons; meaning and measurement.* Human Science Press, New York.
5. Pearce, S. M., Hall, J. F. and Hamblin, G. (1979). *The quality of life of the elderly in residential care: a feasibility study of the development of survey methods.* Polytechnic of North London Survey Research Unit.
6. Armstrong, L. M. (1985). Just alive, or living. *Journal of the American Medical Association*, 253: 789.
7. Schipper, H. (1983). Why measure quality of life? (Editorial). *Canadian Medical Association Journal*, 128: 1367–70.
8. Pearlman, R. A. and Jonsen, A. (1985). The use of quality-of-life considerations in medical decision making. *Journal of the American Geriatric Society*. 33: 344–52.
9. Wilkes, E. (Ed.) (1986). Terminal Care Update Postgraduate Centre Series. Up-date Siebert Publications, Surrey.
10. Wilkes, E. (1984). Dying Now, *Lancet*, i: 950–52.
11. Young, P. (1987). An experiment in long-stay care in hospital. *Geriatric Nursing and Home Care*. 7(1): 26–8.
12. Walden, C. and Norman, A. (1981). Bolingbroke Hospital. Design for decency. *Design for Special Needs*, 42: 11–13.
13. Editorial (1982). The elderly in Denmark: demographic, economic, social and health conditions. *Danish Medical Bulletin*, 29: 89–168.
14. Editorial (1982). A happier old age in Denmark. *British Medical Journal*, 284: 1729–30.
15. Larder, D., Day, P. and Klein, R. (1986). *Pricing the nursing home industry capital and turnover.* University Centre for the Analysis of Social Policy, Bath.
16. Bartlett, H. (1984). The nursing home bonanza. *Health and Social Services Journal*, 4907: 888–9.
17. Ramsay, F., Horsfall, R. and Rudd, A. (1987). Selection for long-term hospital care. *Age and Ageing*, 16: 301–4.

18. Holden, U. and Woods, R. (1982). *Reality Orientation: psychological approaches to the confused elderly.* Churchill Livingstone, Edinburgh..
19. Gurland, B. J. and Cross, P. S. (1982). Epidemiology of psychopathology in old age. Some implications for clinical services. *Psychiatric Clinic of North America*, 5: 11–26.
20. Small, G. W. and Jarvik, L. E. (1982). The Dementia Syndrome. *The Lancet*, ii: 1443–6.
21. Tomlinson, B. E., Blessed, G., and Roth, M. (1970). Observations on the brains of demented old people. *Journal of Neurological Science*, 11: 205–42.
22. Van der Cammen, T. J. M., Simpson, J. M., Fraser, R. M. *et al.* (1987). The Memory Clinic: a new approach to the detection of dementia. *British Journal of Psychiatry*, 150: 359–60.
23. Reisberg, B., Ferris, S. H., de Leon, M. J. and Crook, T. (1982). The global deterioration scale for assessment of primary degenerative dementia. *American Journal of Psychiatry*, 139: 1136–9.
24. Reisberg, B. (1986). Dementia: A systematic approach to identifying reversible causes. *Geriatrics*, 41: 30–46.
25. Jennett, B., Teasdale, G., Fry, J. *et al.* (1980). Treatment for severe head injury. *Journal of Neurology and Neurosurgery*, 43: 289–95.
26. Engelhardt, H. T. and Rie, M. A. (1986). Intensive care units scarce resources and conflicting principles of justice. *Journal of the American Medical Association*, 225: 1159–64.
27. Morgan, C. J. and Braithwaite, M. A. (1986). Severity scoring in intensive care. *British Medical Journal*, 292: 1546.
28. Wagner, A. (1984). Cardiopulmonary resuscitation in the aged. A prospective study. *New England Journal of Medicine*, 310: 1129–30.
29. Zimmerman, J. E., Knaus, W. A., Sharpe, S. M. *et al.* (1986). The uses and implications of Do Not Resuscitate orders in intensive care. *Journal of the American Medical Association*, 255: 351–6.
30. Editorial (1983). Should dying be a diagnosis? *Lancet*, ii: 261.
31. Baskett, P. J. F. (1986) The Ethics of Resuscitation. *British Medical Journal*, 292: 189–90.
32. Lo, B. and Dornbrand, L. (1984). Guiding the hand that feeds. Caring for the demented elderly. *New England Journal of Medicine*, 311: 402–4.
33. Scrutton, S. (1986). Personal effects. *Social Services Insight.* 1(27): 14–15.

3 The Ethical and Legal Framework

Introduction

The ethical and legal principles applicable to the three groups of patients described in Chapter 2 do not differ apart from some statutory intervention in specific cases. However, at least potentially, the outcome of their application may differ between the categories, as indeed they may in relation to different patients within a given category. Much will inevitably depend on the facts of the individual case.

Therefore, in this chapter we discuss the ethical and legal framework within which good medical practice must operate. We look in turn at the notions of competence and incompetence and explore a doctor's ethical and legal obligations when treating patients in the relevant three groups. In the context of the incompetent patient we specifically examine the legal authority, if any, of persons other than the patient to consent to treatment on the patient's behalf and the relevance of an incompetent patient's wishes on the treatment, expressed at a time prior to his incompetence.

The notion of competence

As we shall see, ethical and legal principles differentiate between a patient who is *competent* to make a medical decision on his own behalf and one who is *incompetent* to do so. It is therefore essential to establish at this stage the definitions of these terms — both of which are difficult to spell out and which are often even more difficult to apply to the facts of individual cases.

It is necessary to distinguish between the *concept* of competence and the *criteria* for determining, in a given case, whether the patient is or is not competent. It is important to understand that competence is not a label which may be universally applied to a particular patient since competence is decision-specific. That is, a patient may be competent to reach decision X but not decision Y.

What then is the concept of competence? In English law, it has recently been examined in relation to children and in particular, the extent to which children may be competent to consent to medical treatment upon themselves. The law recognises two elements.[1] Firstly, the individual must possess the ability to understand what is involved in a particular treatment or non-treatment. In other words, the patient must have 'sufficient understanding and intelligence' to comprehend the nature, purpose and likely consequences of undergoing or refusing the treatment. In the situation with which we are concerned in this report, one American case stated that the patient must have the 'ability to understand that in rejecting the (treatment) she is, in effect, choosing death over life'.[2] In addition to having the capacity to understand, the patient must be able to communicate to the physician his or her decision in relation to the particular treatment.

The determination of competence or incompetence is crucial to the way in which the patient is handled by the physician and the extent (if any) of the patient's involvement in the decision-making process. The determination of competence must *prima facie* be for the physician since he is the person dealing with the patient. Although theoretically a court could, with hindsight, say he was wrong in his assessment, this is very unlikely where he made a *bona fide* assessment of the patient's competence. It need hardly be stated that physicians should therefore act with integrity in making this decision and should have regard only to those matters (or criteria) which are relevant to an assessment of competence. In other words, the physician should not strive to deprive the competent patient of his right to choose by disregarding his wishes on the basis of a misplaced view of beneficence or paternalism which leads him to wrongly view the patient as incompetent.

What are the *criteria* for determining competence? It should be remembered that the physician should always be aware of the real possibility that a patient's values and goals may differ from his and so should not necessarily evaluate an unreasonable or potentially damaging decision by the patient as stemming from an incompetent lack of understanding. A mere difference of opinion between a doctor and patient, even if the decision is regarded as unreasonable, should not in itself lead to a finding of incompetence. As one judge put it, a patient has 'a right to decline operative investigation or treatment however unreasonable or foolish this may appear in the eyes of his medical advisers'.[3] The patient 'has a right to be wrong'.[4] Unreasonableness may be *a* factor in assessing lack of understanding but it is not in itself *the* criterion for determining it.

Equally, the physician should not strive to regard an *irrational* decision as incompetently based. Again values and goals may differ. Providing the patient is able to make a thoughtful decision, the patient should not be regarded as incompetent. In one American case a 60-year-old patient diagnosed as schizophrenic, refused a biopsy for suspected breast cancer because she feared the procedure would kill her or interfere with her child-bearing capacity and ability to be a film star. The court examined the patient and found that she understood the possible consequences of her refusal and that she was motivated by the fear of surgery. Even though the court considered this to be 'irrational and foolish', it recognised that the patient was legally competent to refuse treatment.[5]

Nevertheless, a permanently deluded patient may be regarded as incompetent since he or she is not applying values leading to goals which may legitimately differ in society but rather is applying them in a case where he or she is unable to understand what is involved. So, if a patient is unwilling to accept that anything is wrong despite obvious clinical evidence – an example would be gangrene of a limb requiring surgical amputation – then the physician may be justified in regarding the patient as incompetent.[6]

Legal principles

Good medical practice in the treatment of the patients with whom we are concerned in this report must conform to that permitted by law. The legal authorities, either case law or statute, in this area are few and far between. However, general principles and approaches can be detected in the law and stated with some precision, although their precise application to a given case may well be a matter of some uncertainty. Furthermore, the ethical principles of respect for autonomy, beneficence and non-maleficence may assist in determining and explaining the law.

In this report we are primarily concerned with the situation of the incompetent patient and, in particular, the legal effect of his pre-incompetence wishes concerning medical treatment. One way of beginning to establish what is the law, is to examine the relevance of a *competent* patient's wishes in respect of treatment.

The competent patient

The law reflects the ethical principle of respect for another's autonomy in requiring consent to treatment and conversely the right to refuse treatment. A *competent* patient is entitled to refuse treatment since his consent is essential to any treatment which involves an intentional touching of the patient. In the absence of consent the intentional touching will be unlawful, amounting to the tort of battery.[7]

A competent patient should legally be able to refuse *any* medical treatment, including life-saving treatment. There are, however, some criminal law cases which suggest that a doctor may legally override a patient's competently expressed wish not to receive such treatment (*Stone*[8] and *Leigh* v. *Gladstone*[9]). The effect of these cases is far from clear and they have been subjected to considerable criticism.[10,11] It would not be safe (nor sensible) to regard these cases as imposing a duty upon a doctor to save the life of a competent patient against the patient's wishes. At best they may reflect the law's reluctance to punish and impose a penalty upon a doctor who does intervene in such circumstances out of a sense of beneficence.[12]

Two points are worth noting. First, *Stone* was not a case involving a doctor. It concerned the duty of two elderly relatives who had undertaken responsibility for the care of the deceased. It is quite possible that the court regarded the deceased as *incompetent* to refuse treatment because, given her age and condition, she lacked understanding of what was involved in her refusal. Legally, therefore, her wishes in refusing treatment had no effect.[13] Secondly, the case of *Leigh* v. *Gladstone* should be restricted today (if it is the law at all) to the very special circumstances in the case of a prisoner subject to a prison regime refusing food.[14,15]

However, there may be a number of legal limitations upon the right to refuse medical intervention. The extent of these limitations is unclear. Each is based upon the law's view of public policy and what it requires. The most significant limitation concerns the maintenance of public health. While a competent patient's refusal of aggressive intervention must be respected, his refusal of nursing care and other ancillary procedures relating to hygiene may not be. It is probably the case that the law would regard these as a permissible, perhaps even mandatory, basic minimum of providing care in the environment of a hospital or nursing home.

A difficult and complex situation which is interrelated with the obligation to provide 'nursing care', is the ability of a competent patient to refuse artificial nutrition and hydration. One particular difficulty concerns the often made assertion that in such cases the doctor must continue even in the face of a competent refusal because he would otherwise commit the criminal offence of 'counselling or procuring or aiding and abetting suicide' contrary to Section 2 of the Suicide Act 1961. In principle, we believe that a patient is entitled to refuse these interventions, as with any other form of treatment, even if death is the inevitable outcome. We would base our view upon two premises. Firstly, artificial nutrition and hydration should be seen as a form of aggressive intervention and thus subject to the same principles as any other medical interventions which go beyond basic nursing care. This is consistent with recent considered and authoritative opinions on both sides of the Atlantic.[16,17,18] Secondly, we reject the view that in withdrawing or withholding artificial nutrition or hydration the physician assists suicide. We take the view that even if the patient is not suffering from terminal illness from which he would otherwise die, starvation is not suicide. The patient must *positively* do something to himself before his conduct would be so regarded.

Furthermore, even if the law were to regard the patient as committing suicide, the doctor's *omission* to continue artificial feeding or hydration would not be regarded as 'assistance'. This follows either because he must *act* to commit the offence and not merely omit to do something, or because the patient's refusal absolves him of any duty in law to continue treatment.[19,20]

The recent decision of the Court of Appeals in California in *Bouvia*[21] supports this view. The court upheld the right of a competent patient suffering from cerebral palsy with a life expectancy of 15–20 years to refuse tubal feeding. The court recognised that there was a fundamental right to refuse even if the result was to create a 'life-threatening condition' in a patient whose death would not otherwise be imminent. The court affirmed that the decision to refuse was not for the physicians but was 'a moral and philosophical decision that, being a competent adult, is hers alone'. The court considered it 'incongruous, if not monstrous, for medical practitioners to assert their right to preserve a life that someone else must live, or, more accurately, endure, for 15 or 20 years. We cannot conceive it to be the policy of this state to inflict such an ordeal upon anyone'.

While United States law in this area is heavily dependent upon constitutional rights, particularly the right of privacy, we believe English law would reflect the approach of the *Bouvia* case basing itself upon the need for consent to treat which is itself based upon the ethical obligation to respect the individual's autonomy (the leading American decision concerning an *incompetent* patient based its conclusion upon the common law as well as upon constitutional rights: *in re Conroy*[22]).

Even if a court were (wrongly) to regard the refusal of life sustaining procedures as suicide, the physician could not rely upon the once accepted argument that it was justified to use force or act without the consent of the patient to continue or commence treatment or feeding as a reasonable means of preventing a crime (Section 3, Criminal Law Act 1967), since suicide, or attempted suicide, are no longer criminal offences (Section 1, Suicide Act 1961).

We are aware that a series of civil cases[23,24] held that a doctor would, in certain circumstances, be under a duty to prevent the suicide of his patient and would be liable in damages for failure to do so. However, we take the view that these cases should only be applied to *incompetent* patients who are, by definition, unable to act autonomously or, alternatively, they are unlikely to be followed today.[25]

Legal and ethical principle dictates respect for a competent patient's wishes if the physician is certain that the patient holds these wishes. It would be justified in law to seek to obtain evidence of the patient's wishes, but once the physician was satisfied that the patient had refused treatment then no further intervention would be lawful, in our view. As with the assessment of competence, a physician is required to act with integrity and should not out of a misplaced sense of paternalism lean towards the view that the patient's wishes are not clear.

Beyond the need for consent for treatment, a physician's legal obligations (his duty) will be the same as they would be towards any *incompetent* patient. It is to that type of patient, which is the primary concern of our report, that we now turn.

The incompetent patient

When caring for an *incompetent* patient in one of the three categories with which we are concerned, a physician must seek answers to a number of difficult legal questions. Firstly, is there anyone or any institution with the authority to consent to (or refuse) treatment on behalf of the patient who is incapable of consenting for himself? Secondly, is he either permitted or required to act in accordance with the wishes of the patient, expressed prior to his incompetence? If so, can these wishes be expressed informally or must they be contained in a more formal document such as a living will? Thirdly, if there is no-one to consent to (or refuse) treatment and the patient's wishes are unknown or legally irrelevant, what obligations does he owe his patient? We now address each of these in turn.

Consent to (or refusal of) treatment by another

In English law a parent may consent to (or refuse) treatment on behalf of a child who is incompetent because he lacks sufficient intelligence or understanding of the nature and consequences of the medical procedure (*Gillick (supra)*). However, this power is always subject to the Court's *parens patriae* jurisdiction in wardship when the court may overrule a parent's decision and authorise treatment (as in *re B*[26]) or withhold treatment (as in *re D*[27]) according to the court's view of what is required in the best interests of the child.

Outside the parent–child relationship, in English law there is no inherent power in one adult to give consent (or refuse it) on behalf of another (though this is now subject to the revised view of *parens patriae* discussed below). This applies equally to spouses and close relatives.[28] The medical practice of seeking the consent of near relatives, such as spouses or adult children may nevertheless, make good practical sense.

Although there is no common law power to consent to or refuse treatment on behalf of another, there are statutory provisions which entitle (or, arguably do so) physicians to treat certain adults who come within one or more of the relevant categories of patients with which we are concerned. Three main provisions warrant attention:

(1) Mentally disordered persons who are 'liable to be detained', i.e. to be held compulsorily under the Mental Health

Act 1983, may be treated without their consent in accordance with Part 4 of the Act. These provisions do not apply to informal patients since they are not 'liable to be detained' under the Act. If a person falls within the ambit of Part 4 of the Act then he may not be treated other than in accordance with the terms of the Act.[29] However, if the patient does not fall within Part 4 then any authority to treat must be derived from the common law doctrine of necessity based upon public policy, to which we shall return shortly. For example, the 1983 Act only deals with treatment for the patient's mental disorder (Section 63). Treatment for any other illness or injury is not dealt with by the Act (on the provisions of the Act see Gostin[30]).

(2) It might be argued that the guardianship provisions of the 1983 Act (Sections 7–10) offer a solution. However, these only allow a guardian to require a patient to attend a specific place at a particular time for medical treatment. Section 34(1) of the Mental Health Act 1959 went further and, *inter alia*, conferred upon guardians' power to consent to treatment, but this was repealed by Section 8 of the Mental Health (Amendment) Act 1982 and this is reflected in the 1983 Act.

(3) The National Assistance Act 1948 permits a court to make an order under Section 47 to remove a person to a suitable place in order to secure for him 'necessary care and attention'. The section applies to a person (i) who is suffering from grave chronic disease or, being aged, infirm or physically incapacitated and who is living in insanitary conditions and (ii) who is unable to devote to himself – and who is not receiving from other persons – proper care and attention, and (iii) whose removal from home is necessary either in his own interests or for preventing injury to the health of, or serious nuisance to, other persons.

It is unclear whether provisions of 'necessary care and attention' includes medical treatment.[31] In view of the fact that the courts are reluctant to read powers into statutes, especially permitting treatment without consent, it would be unwise to assume Section 47 applies to any person with whom we are concerned who is in need of medical treatment.

As we have observed in the case of minors the court's *parens patriae* wardship jurisdiction allows the court to make decisions, including decisions concerning treatment, on behalf of incompetent children. Does a similar power exist in relation to incompetent adults?

Until recently it had generally been assumed that no such power existed. It seems to be clear that the powers of the Court of Protection under Section 95 of the Mental Health Act 1983, to act 'with respect to the property and affairs of a patient' do not apply to the 'management or care of the patient's body' but are restricted to his financial and property affairs.[32]

However, it now seems that the English courts *may* retain a residuary inherent power to control, *inter alia*, the person of an incompetent adult. In the recent Supreme Court decision in Canada of *Eve*[33] the Court analysed the nineteenth century English cases and recognised the existence of the ancient prerogative *parens patriae* jurisdiction of the Crown over lunatics and those of unsound mind. This jurisdiction 'belong[ed] to the king as *parens patriae*, having the care of those who are not able to take care of themselves, and is founded on the obvious necessity that the law should place somewhere the case of individuals who cannot take care of themselves'.[34] The *Eve* court recognised that this was the original *parens patriae* jurisdiction out of which had grown the now well accepted and often used wardship jurisdiction. The court accepted that the jurisdiction should be exercised on similar principles to wardship. Although there was no case in point, it could be used to authorise *therapeutic* treatment but it could not be used to authorise *non-therapeutic* procedures since this would never be consistent with the underlying basis of the jurisdiction, namely to act for the protection and benefit of the individual.

In *re B (a minor) (wardship: sterilisation)*,[35] the House of Lords was concerned with the court's power to authorise a sterilisation operation on a 17-year-old girl. Although, therefore, the case was one of wardship, the House of Lords made some observations on the existence of the *parens patriae* power in the case of adults. None of the judges explicitly recognised its existence but, equally, none was prepared without much fuller argument to deny its existence. Lord Oliver was content for the purposes of the case to *assume* it existed. Lord Hailsham regarded the reasoning of the Canadian Supreme Court in *Eve* as persuasive.

More recently, in *T* v *T*[36] an English court was, for the first time, asked to acknowledge the existence of the *parens patriae* power in the case of an adult incompetent. In *T* v. *T* the incompetent was a pregnant woman who it was considered ought to undergo an abortion and sterilisation operation, in 'her best interests'. Wood J. accepted, in principle, that the court has a power akin to wardship which it could exercise over incompetent adults, but that it was an *inherent* power of the Crown and not of the court. It was essential, therefore, for the Crown to vest in the Court by warrant under the Sign Manual its *parens patriae* power. Wood J. observed that the last warrant to do this had been revoked in 1960 when the Mental Health Act 1959 came into force. Consequently he held that until such a warrant was made, the power could not be exercised by the court.

Apart then from this technical procedural point, the remaining question must be whether the Mental Health legislation dating from 1960 has superseded and replaced the *parens patriae* jurisdiction in England. It clearly has done in relation to the property and financial affairs of the incompetent mentally ill person but, as we have seen, the 1983 Act does not permit the Court of Protection to authorise medical treatment. It is, therefore, possible that in an appropriate case the court may accept the continued existence of the *parens patriae* jurisdiction in this area (Heywood and Massey[37] and *Eve (supra)*).

The scope of this jurisdiction will approximate to that of wardship and as *re B (supra)* and *re D (supra)* illustrate the court will act according to what it perceived to be the 'best interests' of the patient. It is likely that a court would be cautious in permitting the withdrawal of treatment from an incompetent patient which will result in his death. Nevertheless, such action has been authorised in the United States courts where the *parens patriae* jurisdiction over adult incompetence has long been accepted (*in re Quinlan*[38] and *in re Conroy (supra)*). The scope of this jurisdiction will be examined shortly. In the absence of an authorised third party to give or refuse consent to treatment or an order of the court under its *parens patriae* jurisdiction, a doctor may still be able to treat or withhold treatment from the patient. He will be protected in law by a justification or defence based upon public policy, sometimes called the 'defence of necessity' in those circumstances in which it is thought proper for him to act or withhold treatment. It is the scope of this justification and his legal obligations which are crucial.

Patient wishes

To what extent must a doctor abide by an incompetent patient's earlier expressed wishes? As a matter of principle, clearly expressed wishes should be respected. 'If the patient has foreseen the circumstances which have since arisen and there is no reason to believe that he would have changed his mind if still capable of doing so, the doctor should only be justified in proceeding to the same extent as he could if the patient were still capable of consenting.'[39]

We believe that this statement represents in essence the English law. The extent of intervention contrary to clearly expressed wishes will, as we have seen, be extremely circumscribed. The wishes may be oral or in writing, whether or not in the form of the emerging living will documents. English law in conceding this opportunity to the patient pays due respect to the patient's right of self-determination. It would, in our view, be wrongly paternalistic for a physician to impose his own views upon an incompetent patient who could have lawfully refused the treatment whilst competent.

There is, we concede, no English authority supporting our view of the law. It may therefore be desirable to enact legislation to clarify the law for the avoidance of doubt. Nevertheless, we are confident that this is the legal position. We have little doubt that the English courts would adopt the emerging position in the United States exemplified in the New Jersey Supreme Court decision in *in re Conroy* *(supra)*. We take some time to describe this case because we regard it of crucial significance in the development of English law.

Conroy, an 85-year-old resident of a nursing home, suffered from arteriosclerotic heart disease, hypertension, diabetes and a gangrenous leg. She was doubly incontinent. She was unable to speak but occasionally reacted to external stimuli. She was expected to die within a year. The court was asked by a nephew who was her only relative and guardian, to authorise the removal of artificial feeding and hydration tubes. The court rejected the view that only in the case of the brain-dead or permanently comatose could treatment be refused on the incompetent's behalf. Instead the court recognised an incompetent's constitutional and common law right to refuse treatment including artificial feeding and hydration. The court took the view that if known the patient's wishes would be determinative. The court approved an approach based upon three tests:

1. *The subjective test*

Recognising that the approach of the law should be to determine and effectuate the decision the patient would have made if competent, the court stated that if there was clear evidence that the patient would have refused particular treatment then it would be unlawful to continue when the patient became incompetent.

The court stated that these views might be expressed orally or in a living will, the patient's reaction to medical treatment administered to others, could be deduced from her religious beliefs or from previous conduct in relation to other personal medical decisions.

The court saw no objection to withholding treatment in these circumstances and refused to classify the situation as one of suicide; the cause of death would be the underlying medical condition (cf. *Bouvia* (*supra*) where there is no underlying condition).

2. *Limited-objective test*

In the absence of such clear evidence of the patient's wishes necessary for the 'subjective test', the court held that if there was some 'trustworthy evidence' albeit not 'unequivocally expressed', then treatment could be withheld if the burdens of the treatment in pain and suffering outweigh the benefits to the patient. The court limited this case to a terminally ill patient who is expected to die within a year.

3. *Pure-objective test*

In the absence of any evidence of the patient's wishes, treatment could be withheld only if it would 'clearly and markedly out-weigh the benefits the patient derives from life'. The court determined that any recurring, unavoidable and severe pain which the patient suffers with the treatment should be a reason for withholding it since the administration of the treatment would be inhumane. The *Conroy* court observed that if the court is in any doubt 'it is best to err . . . in favour of preserving life'.

We believe that the approach of the *Conroy* court represents English law, not only on the relevance of the incompetent's earlier wishes but also in the approach to be adopted in their absence even though many of the procedural aspects are inappropriate.

Absence of patient wishes

Although apparently not strictly within the terms of this report, we turn now to the situation where the patient's wishes are unknown. We do so not only because we detect considerable confusion on the part of doctors, but also because the law stated here reflects and gives effect to an ethical framework for medical practice within which all of the problems we are considering fall to be analysed.

In the absence of any known wishes may a physician treat or withhold treatment from a patient? English law recognises a legal justification for treating an incompetent patient where it is *necessary* and *reasonable* to preserve or protect the patient's life or health.[40,41] Short-term incapacity will render fewer procedures necessary than would be the case in a long-term, perhaps permanent, mental incapacity.

Similarly, English law recognises that a physician has a legal justification in changing from treatment for living to treatment for dying for an incompetent patient, as discussed below. English law and medical ethics distinguish between *acts* and *omissions*.[42]

A physician may not intentionally do any act the effect of which is to cause or accelerate the death of the patient. To do so would amount to the very serious criminal offence of murder. Nor, as we have seen, may he knowingly do any act which assists a patient to kill himself.

Nevertheless, moral principle and legal theory recognise that an act done with a good intention (such as the administration of pain-killing drugs) which has an incidental evil effect (accelerating death) is justified.[43] The doctrine of 'double-effect' is now well accepted.[44,45] A doctor who gives on medical grounds increasing doses of a drug to relieve the pain of a terminal cancer patient, even though those doses are such that they in themselves will kill the patient, will not be guilty of murder since his primary intention is the lawful purpose of relieving pain.

However, it is in the realm of withholding or withdrawing life-supporting treatment that the greatest practical difficulties arise and these are reflected in the opaque legal position. Lord Hailsham once stated that 'if you have got a living body, you have got to keep it alive, if you can'.[46] Neither good medical ethics nor legal principle would reach such a result.[47,48] The difficult legal question is to ascertain what precisely are a doctor's obligations in order to determine what he has to do and what he cannot do.

A commonly adopted ethical distinction is between 'ordinary' and 'extraordinary' means. The former are obligatory whilst the latter may be withheld. 'Ordinary' means are 'all medicines, treatments and operations which offer a reasonable hope of benefit for the patient and which can be obtained and used without excessive expense, pain or other inconvenience'. On the other hand 'extraordinary' means are 'all medicines, treatments and operations which cannot be obtained or used without excessive expense, pain or other inconvenience, or which, if used, would not offer a reasonable hope of benefit'.[49,50]

Although in general we agree with this statement of the ethical position and regard it as representing the law, we find the terminology unhelpful. The terms 'ordinary' and 'extraordinary' are often (wrongly) confused with 'common' and 'unusual' procedures which look not to their effect upon the patient but to the level of utilisation at a particular time by the medical profession. In other words, if this distinction is applied, today's 'extraordinary' treatment may become tomorrow's 'ordinary' treatment. For example, antibiotics would at one time have been an 'unusual' treatment. Today no-one could argue for such a view. Yet, morally we consider that in some cases a doctor would be justified in withholding antibiotics from an incompetent and terminally ill patient whose pain and suffering would merely be continued for a short period prior to the patient's inevitable death.

An equally misleading misunderstanding of the term turns upon the difference between elaborate technological interventions ('extraordinary') and more common place and simpler medical procedures ('ordinary').

Apart from the obvious difficulties of applying this and the earlier distinction, we believe both interpretations of the terms are inappropriate since they are *without moral significance* and, we would suggest, *without legal significance*.[51] They portray the 'extraordinary'/'ordinary' dichotomy as merely *descriptive* when, in truth, it is a *normative* test based upon a balance of benefits and burdens. Its application 'depends on whether it is a good thing for the life to be prolonged'.[52]

Thus, along with other commentators, we consider it unhelpful to adopt the 'extraordinary'/'ordinary' distinction. Indeed, we agree with the suggestion that it is potentially very misleading.[53,54] Instead, we believe that the law would adopt the substance of the proper distinction between the terms but should not utilise the terminology. In essence, this would be in line with the third and objective test proposed by the *Conroy* court. It follows that a doctor's legal obligations would, in our view, be determined in the case of an incompetent patient who had expressed no prior wishes, on the basis of an objective test weighing in the balance the benefits and the burdens of the proposed treatment. In our view, the distinction between unduly burdensome and beneficial treatments is morally determinative and should also be legally conclusive. We quote and rely upon the following passage in the US President's Commission Report, *Deciding to Forego Life-Sustaining Treatment*.[55]

> ... a patient should not have to undergo life-prolonging treatment
> without consideration of the burdens that the treatment would
> impose. Of course, whether a treatment is warranted depends on its
> usefulness or benefit as well. Whether serious burdens of treatment
> (for example, the side effect of chemotherapy treatments for cancer)
> are worth enduring depends on the expected benefits – how long the
> treatment will extend life, and under what conditions. Usefulness
> might be understood as mere extension of life, no matter what the
> condition of that life. . . . Extraordinary treatment is that which, in
> the patient's view, entails significantly greater burdens than benefits
> and is therefore undesirable and not obligatory, while ordinary
> treatment is that which, in the patient's view, produces greater
> benefits than burdens and is therefore reasonably desirable and
> undertaken.

We do not consider that the general position can be stated more clearly than this. We suggest that the benefit/burden balance is, and should be, part of English law.

We note the statement of the President's Commission that the precise position of the balance should be seen from the patient's point of view. We entirely accept this approach as our earlier statements in this chapter indicate. This would clearly be applicable where the court can apply the 'subjective' and 'limited-objective' test in *Conroy*. Otherwise, we take the view that the doctor must do his best, attempting in so far as he is able, to have regard to the patient's circumstances, values and interests to determine the outcome of the benefit/burden test. Ultimately, he must act in the best interests of the patient without seeking to impose his own values upon the patient, whose life (and dying process) is at issue. In the USA, the absence of evidence of a patient's wishes has been interpreted by some doctors as requiring them to exercise maximum medical efforts to maintain the patient's survival. We do not agree with this interpretation.

What medical procedures may a doctor lawfully withhold from his patient? Clearly the medically futile will not be obligatory since the burdens must necessarily outweigh the benefits. However, outside this case the question must fall to be assessed by the doctor. The decision-making role of the doctor in this situation is clearly a difficult one, but providing he is honestly and reasonably exercising his judgement, having regard to the benefits and burdens of treatment in relation to the pain, suffering and likely period of survival of the patient, then we believe a court would consider the doctor to be acting lawfully.

References

1. *Gillick* v. *DHSS* [1986] 1 AC 112.
2. *Lane* v. *Candura* [1978] 576 N.E. 2d 1232, 1236.
3. *Smith* v. *Auckland Hospital Board* [1965] NZLR 191, 219 per Greeson J.
4. *Hopp* v. *Lepp* (1979) 98 DLR (3d) 464, 470 per Prowse J.
5. *In re Yetter* (1973) 62 PA and DLC 2d 619.
6. *State Department of Human Services* v. *Northern* (1978) 563 SW 2d 197.
7. *Murray* v. *McMurray* [1949] 2 DLR 442.
8. *Stone* [1977] QB 354.
9. *Leigh* v. *Gladstone* (1909) 26 TLR 139.
10. Kennedy [1976] The Legal Effect of Requests by the Terminally Ill and Aged not to Receive Further Treatment from Doctors. *Criminal Law Review*, 217–32.
11. Williams, Glanville (1983). *Textbook of Criminal Law*, 2nd edition. Stevens & Sons, London. 262 *et seq*.
12. *Attorney General of British Columbia* v. *Astaforoff* [1984] 4 WWR 385.
13. *Smith* [1979] Criminal Law Review 251.
14. Kennedy, op. cit.
15. Zellick [1976] PL 153.
16. Editorial (1986). Terminal Dehydration. *Lancet*, 1: 306.
17. Lo, B. and Dornbrand, L. (1984). Guiding the hand that feeds. Caring for the demented elderly. *New England Journal of Medicine*, 311: 402–4.
18. Volicer *et al.* (1986). Hospice approach to the treatment of patients with advanced dementia of the Alzheimer type. *Journal of the American Medical Association*, 256: 2210–13.

19. Kennedy, op. cit.
20. Williams, G. L. (1973). Euthanasia. *Medico-legal Journal*, **41**: 14–31.
21. *Bouvia* v. *Superior Court of the State of California* (1986) 225 Cal Reptr 297.
22. *In re Conroy* 486 A 2d 1209 [1985].
23. *Selfe* v. *Ilford and District HMC* (1970) 114 Solicitors Journal 935.
24. *Thorne* v. *Northern Group HMC* (1964) 108 Solicitors Journal 484.
25. For example *Hyde* v. *Tameside AHA*. The Times, 16 April 1981.
26. *Re B (a minor)* [1981] 1 WLR 1421.
27. *Re D (a minor)* [1976] Fam 185.
28. Skegg, P. D. G. (1984). *Law, Ethics and Medicine*, p. 72. Clarendon Press, Oxford.
29. *R* v. *Hallstrom ex p W* [1986] 2 All ER 306.
30. Gostin, L. (1986). *Mental Health Services – Law and Practice*, Chapter 20. Shaw & Sons, London.
31. Hoggett, B. (1984), *Mental Health Law*, 2nd edition. Sweet and Maxwell, London.
32. *Re W (EEM)* [1971] Ch. 123, 143 per Ungoed-Thomas J.
33. *Re Eve* [1986] 31 DLR (4th) 1.
34. *Wellesley* v. *Duke of Beaufort* (1987) 38 ER 236, 243 per Lord Eldon.
35. *Re B (a minor) (wardship: sterilisation)* [1987] 2 All ER 206.
36. *T* v. *T*. [1988] 2 WLR 189.
37. Heywood, N. A. and Massey, A. S. (1978). *Court of Protection Practice*, 10th edition. Stevens & Sons, London.
38. *In re Quinlan* 355 A 2d 647 [1976].
39. Skegg, P. D. G. op. cit. 116.
40. *Marshall* v. *Curry* [1933] 3 DLR 260.
41. Skegg, P. D. G. (1974). A justification for medical procedures performed without consent. *Law Quarterly Review*, **90**: 512–30.
42. See for example Gillon, R. (1986). *Philosophical Medical Ethics*, Chapter 20. John Wiley & Sons, Chichester.
43. *Bodkin Adams* [1957] Criminal Law Review 365.
44. Gillon R., op. cit. Chapter 21.
45. *Arthur* (1981) 78 Law Society Gazette 1341 per Farquharson J.
46. *The Listener*, 8 July 1976.
47. Gillon R., op. cit. Chapters 20 and 22.
48. Skegg, P. D. G. (1984). *Law, Ethics and Medicine*, Chapter 7. Clarendon Press, Oxford.
49. Kelly, G. (1958). *Medico-Moral Problems*, p. 129 The Catholic Hospital Association, St Louis.
50. Ramsey, P. (1970). *The Patient As Person*, p. 122 Yale University Press, New Haven.
51. The President's Commission Report (1983). *Deciding to Forego Life-Sustaining Treatment*, pp. 87–8. US Government Printing Office, Washington D.C.
52. Rachels, J. (1986) *The End of Life*, p. 99. Oxford University Press,

Oxford.
53. Gillon, R., op. cit. Chapter 22.
54. Ramsey, P. (1978). *Ethics at the Edge of Life*, p. 153. Yale University Press, New Haven.
55. The President's Commission Report, op. cit., p. 88.

4 The Possible Role for Advance Directives

The purpose of advance directives

The primary purpose of advance directives is to give effect to a patient's right to refuse or change treatment. Except in an emergency, any medical investigation, treatment or procedure can, as we have seen, only be carried out with the patient's consent. The form of the consent is irrelevant save for evidential purposes, but must be obtained unless there is an unequivocal presumption of consent.

An obvious consequence of this is the implication that if a competent patient refuses consent, no medical action may be taken in the area relating to the refusal. It is of course part of the doctor's responsibility to ensure, insofar as it is possible, that a refusal of treatment is made with a full understanding of the possible consequences. This is especially true in the case of an illness which may be life-threatening without a particular treatment. Doctors have found it difficult to accept this as a patient's right. Much of the doctor's difficulty relates to the question of the patient's competence to make a decision. It is relatively easy to diminish a person's claim to be competent either by asserting that the complexities of the medical considerations are beyond the ability of the person to comprehend, or by arguing that there is a psychiatric disorder such as depression which could distort the person's interpretation of the facts. In these circumstances the doctor may feel he has no option but to employ traditional paternalism which, in varying degrees, has been a feature of the doctor–patient relationship.

Western society has, however, increasingly questioned the role of paternalism, particularly in the USA, and there have been several eloquent pleas for paternalism to be replaced by a partnership of understanding between patient and doctor.[1,2]

The growing background of concern over the limits of medical treatment has given rise to uncertainty on both sides of the doctor–patient relationship. The widening range of therapeutic and technological options in the management of advanced illness may aggravate the medical uncertainties about how far to pursue a policy for living rather than a policy for dying. With the greater numbers of elderly patients with multi-system disease, concern about the quality of a particular life will become more common. Yet, at the same time, the definition and assessment of 'quality of life' have not been fully addressed by doctors and society, and although some progress has been made (see Chapter 2), no agreement is currently in sight.

From the point of view of patients, the growth of medical technology is often associated with an image of medicine striving to preserve life at the expense of individual personal dignity. Even without high-technology medicine, there is some concern that new treatments may encourage doctors to pursue their patients' survival when the lay observer might think the dying process should be left to take its course without intrusion.

Thus, on both sides of the professional relationship there is evidence of growing uncertainty of what can and should happen towards the end of life. The mutual recognition of uncertainty may be one of several forces acting to encourage the broader exchange of value judgements and personal views on life and death between doctors and patients. In this context, advance directives are a means of giving permanent expression to a patient's wishes of how the uncertainty may be shared and managed, even when one partner, the patient, can no longer express his views.

What is not known is whether those who might consider making use of advance directives, if they were available, have an accurate knowledge of the relevant medical conditions, and how they perceive their quality of life should be affected. Before introducing advance directives research would be required on this subject and educational and monitoring programmes developed to ensure their effectiveness in reflecting people's true intentions.

The question has been raised whether some doctors might refuse to act on the provisions of an advance directive, on the grounds that it was against their conscience. They would have no justification for doing so either ethically or legally when the request was to withhold or withdraw treatment, because they would be carrying out treatment without consent. To proceed with such treatment in opposition to the instructions of a legally valid advance directive would therefore constitute a tort of battery, and hence be unlawful.

As has been seen, advance directives have received much attention in the USA. The impetus for change there was generated in large part by the publication in 1983 of the President's Commission Report entitled *Deciding to Forego Life-Sustaining Treatment* (previously cited in Chapter 3). It received wide publicity and led to extensive public debate. It strongly affirmed the supremacy of patient autonomy and commended the wider exchange of information and opinions between doctors and patients. On the matter of advance directives the report states, 'The Commission believes that advance directives are, in general, useful as a means of appropriate decision-making about life-sustaining treatment for incapacitated patients. The education of the general public and of health care professionals should be a concern to legislators, as the statutes are ineffective if unknown or misunderstood' (p. 149).

The benefits of advance directives are said to be the following:

(1) An advance directive is an expression of patient autonomy which for some patients is reassuring, should they suffer from serious permanent illness or disability, or terminal illness.

(2) Completion of an advance directive may alleviate the fear of unbearable pain in terminal malignant disease.

(3) Discussions between patients and doctors on the use of advance directives will create increased medical awareness of anxieties relating to advanced incurable and terminal

disease.

(4) So-called defensive, or over-intrusive medical care is likely to be discouraged by the existence of advance directives.

(5) An advance directive may aid doctors and others confronted with the ethical dilemmas of cancer medicine, intensive care medicine, resuscitation and geriatric medicine.

(6) An advance directive is likely to reduce the level of stress and distress in a patient's relatives.

(7) The arbitrariness of medical decision-making in response to certain ethical dilemmas may be reduced by the use of an advance directive.

Some people have proposed the introduction of advance directives on different grounds, that of saving resources (see Chapter 1). We do not consider this to be an ethically respectable reason for advocating them. We regard respect for the liberty of individuals as paramount, and people should not therefore be pressured into acting in order to save resources. It is the case that the introduction of advance directives would lead to a direct saving of some resources, but the level of such savings is difficult to predict, because it will depend on the numbers of people who sign such directives, the particular provisions they make, and the future state of their health. There is also the likelihood that improvements in the general level of care will accompany the introduction of advance directives and offset any direct savings. The overall effect on resources is therefore impossible to predict with any certainty, and it would be unwise for assumptions about resources to be made in advance.

The legal validity of advance directives

Much of the relevant background has already been discussed in Chapter 3. We have seen that the legal standing of advance directives cannot be stated with certainty, since there is no specific legislation and the issue has never come before an English court.

Living wills

In considering the non-statutory use of living wills we have seen that some cases in the USA suggest that a patient's wishes expressed prior to becoming incompetent may be relevant in guiding a doctor's obligations once the patient has become incompetent.[3,4] In England, the courts could take the same approach so that a doctor might be empowered to withdraw treatment, including life-saving treatment, if that had been the wish of the patient. The issue is not, however, as simply put as this. Analytically, there are two distinct questions to be considered. The first concerns advance directives which contain a request to do that which is at present lawful (as set out in Chapter 3). Here, what is at issue is the legal validity and effect of the request. Secondly, we must consider the quite separate problem of the directive which contains a request to do that which may not be lawful. In this second situation it is the lawfulness of the requested conduct as well as the validity of the request which is at issue.

It is by no means certain that an English court would adopt the view now gaining ground in the USA. It is most likely, given the present state of the law, that an English court would regard the pre-incompetence wishes of the patient as merely *directory* and not as imposing any obligation. The outcome would be that the decision to commence or continue life-sustaining treatment would be a matter for the doctor having regard to his perception of the best interests of the patient. Indeed, any doctor who did intervene would have legal justification if an action were brought by a disgruntled and by now competent patient in relation to such intervention.[5]

Powers of attorney

As regards powers of attorney, under the common law it is arguable that an adult patient could nominate another as his agent so that the other may take decisions concerning the patient's health. There seems, however, to be no reported case in which this has occurred. In any event, any agency would (in the absence of any statutory provision) terminate on the incompetence of the patient.

As for statute law, the agency which a person may create for the management of his affairs under the Powers of Attorney Act 1971, terminates on the incompetence of that person. However, the Enduring Powers of Attorney Act 1985 permits the creation of a power of attorney which, providing certain statutory conditions are met, continues after the creator has become incompetent. Although the Act was designed to give power to deal specifically with the financial affairs of the individual, the question arises whether Section 3(1) of the Act, which states that the scope of the general authority of an enduring power of attorney extends to an incompetent's 'property or affairs', thereby covers health care decisions, specifically about treatment. It is most unlikely that a court would so construe the statute in the light of the treatment of what is now Section 95 of the Mental Health Act 1983 in *re W (EEM)* [1971]. When interpreting the Court of Protection's powers 'with respect to the property and affairs of a patient' in relation to this case Ungoed–Thomas stated that the court did not have jurisdiction over 'the management or care of the patient's person'[6] (see also Chapter 3).

It seems, therefore, that without a specific statutory provision creating an enduring power of attorney in relation to health care decisions, this form of advance directive has no legal validity, unlike (for example) in California, since the Durable Power of Attorney Health Care Act 1983.

The case for legislation governing living wills

An examination of the legal developments in the USA may help to identify the extent to which there is a case for introducing legislation on living wills in the UK. The growth of legislation on living wills in America has been quite remarkable. California adopted its 'Natural Death Act' in 1976, and in the subsequent ten years 38 of the 50 United States introduced similar legislation.

Although the statutes appear under a variety of names (e.g. 'Medical Treatment Decision Act', Arizona; 'Death with Dignity Act', Arkansas; 'Life Prolonging Procedure Act', Florida; 'Living Wills Act', Georgia; 'Life-sustaining Procedures Act', Iowa; 'Withholding or Withdrawal of Life-sustaining Procedures', Nevada; 'Right to Die Act', New Mexico) they are broadly similar. In preparing living wills, nearly all these states require the use of prescribed declaration forms, although these vary between states.

In 1985 the National Conference of Commissioners on Uniform State Laws, which undertakes the drafting of legislation when there is an evident need for conformity within the 50 states, approved a 'Rights of the Terminally Ill' Act. The Commissioners recognised the need to allow the expression of patient autonomy in a uniform way which could be applied throughout the USA. The act was drafted with the help of such groups as the American Hospital Association, the American Bar Association's Commission on Legal Problems of the Elderly, and the Catholic Health Association of the United States. The concept of allowing individuals to express their wishes about a future terminal or life-threatening illness is clearly widely used and commands the support of much of the American medical, legal and religious establishments. The rapid progression of State laws indicates a widespread public demand for appropriate legislation.

In the various State laws on living wills and in the Uniform Rights of the Terminally Ill Act of 1985, there are detailed provisions on such matters as the definition of terminology, immunity from legal liability for doctors who comply with a directive, recording the existence of a living will, methods of revocation, and the protection of benefits under policies of life assurance.

It has been suggested that the next generation of laws on living wills should be strengthened by insisting upon penalties against doctors who fail to conform to written instructions. Nonetheless, it is already evident that the various State laws have had a significant effect on medical practice in the USA. It has been said that the doctor–patient relationship has been changed by the intense legalisation of American medicine,[7] piling external constraints in the form of law on the ethical framework operated by the profession. Because of conflicting and highly public legal judgments, American medical care of patients at the end of life is said by some to be confused and defensive: 'Legal pressures may prompt physicians to ignore death as an ethical right'[8] and, as a consequence, 'our professional code of ethics lacks a coherent, stable, and principled foundation'.[9] By contrast, others have seen the law differently. Recent cases in New York and California have had to fill the vacuum of uncertainty even if, by so doing, they have 'forced seriously ill and dying patients and their grieving families to endure the additional rigours of courtroom litigation in order to win respect for their well-established right as competent adults to decline treatments that prolong the dying process'.[10]

What lesson can be learned for the UK from these developments? It is clear that some action is needed in Britain to give effect to the wishes of competent people concerning how they want to be treated if they become incompetent. Is the American model appropriate or is there an alternative approach? Let us turn to the detailed analysis of how a living will may be executed and what it should contain.

Although in a few of the American states living wills are designed to be signed, witnessed, and put into effect while the patient is still competent, the great majority are aimed at taking effect at some point after the patient has become incompetent. It is this latter form that is envisaged in this report.

As the discussion in previous chapters has shown, both the public and doctors appear to have a clear notion of which medical situations give rise to the commonest and most worrying dilemmas. In the light of this, the challenge posed by living wills is to devise a document which specifically responds to these.

There are three principal prerequisites for making the living will perform its function as a prospective expression of autonomy. They are: (1) the phrasing of a declaration should reflect what the person considers to be the circumstances in which it might be used; (2) these circumstances should be identifiable;

and (3) the recommendations contained in the declaration should be capable of being implemented within the accepted ethical and legal standards of medical practice.

In order to ensure that these prerequisites can be interpreted in a clinical setting the text of a living will should be precisely drafted. Particular attention needs to be directed to the event which will trigger the living will and to the procedures to be carried out when the time for implementation arrives.

In respect of the *triggering event* three alternatives are possible. The trigger can be incompetence alone, or incompetence with the addition of a particular condition or disability, or incompetence with the addition of terminal illness. Each of these definitions gives rise to particular difficulties. Incompetence alone may cause a living will to be implemented in circumstances which some people would consider inappropriate, for example, a moderate degree of dementia without other disability. Incompetence plus specified conditions or disabilities may lead to problems because of the impossibility of itemising every conceivable triggering clinical circumstance, and the uncertainty in interpreting those which are specified. Incompetence plus terminal illness does not capture all the circumstances under which many people would wish a living will to be instituted. It may also cause problems if clinicians interpret terminal illness restrictively, as occurred in the operation of the California Natural Death Act 1976.[11]

Whichever of these definitions is adopted it should be noted that they apply only to people who are permanently incompetent. It is not uncommon for those who are chronically ill, for example, with dementia, to demonstrate fluctuating competence, and it would be both inappropriate and unworkable to attempt to apply advance directives in such circumstances.

In respect of the *procedures to be adopted* once the living will has come into operation, the more vague the declaration, the less reassured might the patient be that his wishes would be met, and the less able might the doctor be to decide whether or when to implement those wishes. Furthermore, imprecise situations might be thought to oblige both patient and doctor to discuss and agree what they thought each other had in mind. This might require lengthy discussion, which could still be inconclusive. Also, if these discussions were not carefully recorded, they could well be ignored, given the high chance that the doctor who had to decide on the issue when the patient was incompetent would not be the same doctor.

These arguments favour detailed specific instructions, but some would take the view that the declared spirit in which the living will is used in the first place allows those responsible for the patient's care sufficient discretion to implement the living will even in those circumstances in which particular disease states are not specifically mentioned. There might also be a conflict for individuals who found it easy and comforting to sign a readily prepared declaration, whilst at the same time wishing to trust the doctor to attend to them as he saw fit, once it came to be implemented. 'The patient ordinarily trusts his physician not only to act in his best interest during his life but also to see that his death is as comfortable, decent and peaceful an event as possible. This is an implied trust that he may not want to verbalise or discuss.'[12] So, equally, there is a counter-argument favouring more general instructions.

Another issue is whether a prescribed form should be used in drawing up a living will. The American Legal Advisors Committee of Concern for Dying proposed a 'Model Act for the Right to Refuse Treatment' in which the following recommendation was made: 'No specific form or document is included because we believe the individuals' wishes will be more likely to be set forth if their own words are used'.[13] This recommendation assumes that people are capable of expressing their wishes unambiguously. The many versions of the living will in the USA are testimony, however, to the fact that even for those experienced in the field, it is not easy to find an appropriate form of words (although there is broad uniformity of sense). A further difficulty arising from allowing complete individual freedom to write a living will is that there may be a considerable gap between the patient's expectations and medical and legal reality. Patients might well make requests for that which would be medically unsound or legally untenable. In such a case, the doctor responsible for implementing the living will may be exposed to ethical and legal insecurity. Whether a prescribed form is advised or not it is recommended that all those preparing living wills are advised to consult with a professional experienced in the field, most probably their own general practitioner or solicitor, before drawing up the document.

There are therefore advantages and disadvantages to having a prescribed form of declaration. On balance, however, such a form is probably desirable. Two *Draft Model Living Will Declaration Forms* are set out below, to illustrate the different approaches which may be adopted.

If the time comes when I am incapacitated to the point when I can no longer actively take part in decisions for my own life, and am unable to direct my physician as to my own medical care, I request that I be allowed to die and not be kept alive through life-sustaining measures if my condition is deemed irreversible. I do not intend any direct taking of my life, but only that my dying not be unreasonably prolonged.

It is my express wish that if I should develop
(a) brain disease of severe degree, or
(b) serious brain damage resulting from accidental or other injury or illness, or
(c) advanced malignant disease,
in which I would be physically unable or mentally incompetent to express my own opinion about accepting or declining treatment, and if two independent physicians conclude that, to the best of current medical knowledge, my condition is irreversible, then I request that the following points be taken into consideration.

(contd)

1. Any separate illness (e.g. pneumonia, or a cardiac or kidney condition) which may threaten my life should not be given active treatment unless it appears to be causing me undue physical suffering. Cardiopulmonary resuscitation should not be used if the existing quality of my life is already seriously impaired.

2. In the course of such an advanced illness, if I should be unable to take food, fluid or medication, I would wish that these should not be given by any artificial means, except for the relief of obvious suffering.

3. If, during any such illness, my condition deteriorates without reversible cause and, as a result, my behaviour becomes violent, noisy, or in other ways degrading, or if I appear to be suffering severe pain, any such symptom should be controlled immediately by appropriate drug treatment, regardless of the consequences upon my physical health and survival, to the extent allowed by the law.

4. Other requests.

The object of this declaration is to minimise distress or indignity which I may suffer or create during an incurable illness, and to spare my medical advisers and/or relatives the burden of making difficult decisions on my behalf.

These two forms represent examples of possible options. The first specifies incompetence as the sole criterion for bringing the living will into operation and does not give directions as to how the person's care should be managed. The second differs in both these respects.

Practical and procedural matters

Some of the practical and procedural matters which might arise in relation to living wills are discussed briefly below.

(a) *Formalities in relation to the elderly*
If it is decided to introduce living wills, it is important to notice that a large proportion of people wishing to have recourse to them are likely to be elderly. Thus, the formalities involved would arguably have to be the bare minimum to establish the document's validity.

(b) *Capacity*
The person making a living will should be a competent adult. Provided competence is defined, the question whether the test is satisfied is a matter for clinical judgment. In the event of a dispute as to whether the person was competent to execute the document, it is suggested that it should be presumed that he was, i.e. the onus of proving that he was not is upon the person so claiming. Alternatively, it could be a requirement that the witnesses (see (c) below) sign a declaration that the person appears to be of sound mind when the instrument is executed.

(c) *Signature and witnesses*
A living will document, whether of a standard type or in the person's own words, would have to be signed and dated by the person making it. It is a uniform requirement of existing legislation on living wills that there should be witnesses, as a safeguard against coercion. It is suggested that there should be two competent adults, one of whom might be the person's family doctor or a hospital consultant in the case of a hospitalised patient.

A question arises as to whether certain persons, such as creditors or potential beneficiaries, should be excluded from witnessing. It is unlikely that creditors would be selected as witnesses. Perhaps the best solution is that at least one witness must be neither a relative nor a person who would take any part of the estate by will or otherwise on the death of the person involved.

(d) Notification and recording
The person making the living will would notify near relatives or friends (if any) of his action, and also his medical practitioner (if not a witness), and legal adviser. The medical practitioner would make a written note in the case records. There would also be a procedure for having the information recorded in any appropriate hospital records.

(e) Availability of blank forms
If prescribed living will declaration forms were to be used, consideration should be given to methods of making blank forms readily available, possibly from doctors' surgeries and hospital wards, and from professional legal advisers.

(f) Notice and implementation
The means whereby a living will might be brought into effect will vary. Provision should be made for ensuring that the existence of a living will is brought to the attention of the doctor (see (d) above). The most common ways of implementing it would probably be as follows:

(i) *The patient.* A seriously ill patient, when still conscious and competent might implement a previously signed living will as a means of substantiating and formalising a request for treatment to be withheld or withdrawn. At a particular juncture in an illness the patient might ask the attending doctors to refer to the living will and to consider implementing it forthwith.

Alternatively, a patient when already gravely ill could request a copy of a living will for signature and subsequent implementation when the circumstances were deemed to be suitable.

 (ii) *A relative or friend.* When a patient has become incompetent and a relative or close friend with knowledge of the patient's living will considered that the time was approaching or had arrived to consider implementing it, an approach could be made to a member of the medical staff.

(iii) *The legal adviser.* If the patient had notified his legal adviser that he had signed a living will form, the legal adviser, either from his own knowledge of the patient's serious condition or by information from others, could suggest to the medical staff that it might be appropriate to implement the living will.

(iv) *The doctor.* The patient's general practitioner or a hospital doctor knowing of a living will in the case records could suggest to the doctor in charge of the patient that the circumstances for implementing the living will might be considered.

 (v) *A nurse, social worker, minister or other person involved in the care of the patient.* Any person with medical knowledge who was aware of the patient's state of health and of the living will could indicate to the medical attendants an opinion that the time might have come to implement the living will.

(g) *Consultation procedure*

When a doctor caring for a patient known to have completed a living will determines (spontaneously or at another's suggestion) that the circumstances might be appropriate to implement the living will, it may be appropriate to notify any next of kin, if possible. If the patient's wishes would be met by implementing the living will and the circumstances were deemed appropriate, it would be advisable to record the relevant facts and opinions in the medical record.

(h) *Revocation*

It is essential to an acceptance of the notion of living wills that it be clear that a person may revoke his living will at any time, by destroying or defacing it, or by asking someone else to do so on his behalf. The living will may also be revoked at any time by verbal or written instructions from the signatory to his doctor, legal adviser, or other responsible person. Any legal or medical records must thereupon be amended to take note of the revocation, and any such alteration should be signed and dated. The execution of a living will should also revoke any earlier instrument.

More problematic is the question of revocation when incompetent. The logical expectation is that an incompetent person cannot revoke, as in the case of ordinary wills, for example. However, most of the American legislation permits revocation even after loss of competence. Although at first sight this seems to defeat the object of the exercise, the point is that it would be invidious to refuse treatment which the patient, although confused, is at present requesting. This is a strong argument for accepting revocation despite the person's incompetence. Even if it is thought that the person should only be able to revoke while competent, it should be presumed that he was competent at the time of revocation, so that the onus of proving the contrary is on the person so claiming.

(i) *Time limits*

Should a living will lapse after a specified number of years? On the one hand it might be undesirable if the person's fate should be determined by means of an instrument executed decades ago and now forgotten, while on the other hand the person may fail to recognise the passing of a time limit and therefore fail to reconsider the matter. It would clearly be desirable that the provisions of a living will should be reviewed on a regular basis, perhaps every five or ten years. People completing living wills should therefore be advised accordingly, but to make this mandatory would be administratively complex and costly and some people might prefer not to undertake such review at specified times. Therefore it is thought that, on balance, it is better that no obligatory review or time limit is imposed.

(j) *Liability*

A doctor who reasonably and in good faith and after appropriate consultation, acted upon a living will would not be exposed to subsequent civil liability or criminal prosecution. Further, no question of professional misconduct would arise in such circumstances.

If the doctor deliberately disregards the instructions of a living will, consideration should be given as to what if any sanctions should apply and to whether these should ge beyond professional censure.

Recourse to fraud, forgery, concealment or destruction in the preparation or implementation of a living will would clearly attract appropriate criminal liability.

(k) *Life assurance*

It would be necessary to make it clear as a matter of law, whether by agreement with assurance companies or by legislation, that the completion or implementation of a living will was to have no effect upon the terms of an existing life assurance policy, particularly as regards any provision excluding cover in the case of suicide (i.e. execution of a living will and then compliance by others with its terms do not amount to suicide).

(l) *Pregnancy*

If a living will comes into operation in relation to a woman who is pregnant, any instructions to forego life-sustaining treatment should be regarded as invalid during the course of the pregnancy.

The case for durable powers of attorney

Introduction

We have already examined the question whether a living will declaration or a durable power of attorney for health care decisions have any validity under the present law. As far as durable powers of attorney are concerned, it was concluded (in contrast to the views expressed in the President's Commission Report concerning similar statutes in the USA[14]) that they probably did not fall within the Enduring Powers of Attorney Act 1985 (in which case they could not be effective, as there is no other way in which a power of attorney can survive the incompetence of the principal). Even if they did come within the 1985 Act, amendments would be required in order to provide the safeguards which would be necessary to the use of a power of attorney in the context of health care decision-making. The discussion which follows proceeds upon two assumptions:

(1) that the present law makes no provision, or no satisfactory provision, for the use of a power of attorney in respect of health care decisions after the principal has become incompetent; and
(2) that the law should provide for the implementation of a person's instructions, given while competent, as to his medical treatment in the event of supervening incompetence.

Living wills and durable powers of attorney compared

Experience in the United States with living will legislation has resulted in recommendations that the goal of patient autonomy would be more effectively achieved if the law provided for durable powers of attorney for health care decision-making, either as an alternative to a living will declaration or in combination with such a declaration. (See the President's Commission Report[15] and the conclusions of the Legal Advisors Committee of Concern for Dying.[16]) What follows is an attempt to summarise the respective advantages and disadvantages of living wills and durable powers of attorney, with a view to establishing how the desired objective can best be achieved.

(a) *Drafting problems*
Existing examples of living will legislation seem to suffer from unsatisfactory drafting. The problem is to strike a balance

between terms which are too general and those which are too specific. If the declaration is too general, it might fail to achieve the goal of patient autonomy because a large measure of discretion will inevitably be left with the doctor. If it is too specific, it may not deal with the particular problem which arises. While the drafting could be improved, it seems inevitable that the durable power of attorney must be more advantageous in this respect. Whatever criterion governs the agent's decision-making (this is discussed on pages 70–1), the point is that he will make his decision in the light of the actual circumstances at the time the question arises. Hence a durable power of attorney, or a durable power combined with a living will declaration, must be preferable in this respect to a living will alone.

(b) *Non-medical considerations*
Of less importance, but not entirely without significance, is the question whether non-medical matters can play any part in the decision process. The timing of death can have financial consequences, for example, in the tax context. A living will is unlikely to permit such considerations to be taken into account. This raises the issue of whether the doctor can take such matters into consideration in a case involving no living will or durable power of attorney. For example, would the doctor be acting in the patient's interests if he kept him alive until a particular date for tax reasons, or until a relative gets married or arrives from Australia? To the extent that the doctor could take non-medical matters into account, then a person acting under a power of attorney should also be entitled to do so. In the absence of express provision, however, the point remains unclear. This is a matter which would affect only a small minority of patients, but some consideration should be given to the problem.

(c) *Abuse*
There is always a possibility that a person's free will may be overborne by the exercise of undue influence or pressure. This is so whatever the nature of the transaction, whether it is a

living will, an ordinary will, a durable power of attorney or any other power of attorney. As far as contracts, gifts and other dispositions are concerned, the law deals with the problem by allowing the transaction to be set aside in certain circumstances. The requirements of writing, signature and witnesses are directed to minimising the possibility of undue pressure, and are a feature of wills, living wills and powers of attorney. It is not thought that a durable power of attorney is either more or less inherently liable to abuse in this respect.

However, one possible disadvantage of the durable power of attorney is that there is a possibility of abuse at the later stage, when the decision is made. It is not suggested that the agent is likely to act deliberately in bad faith. (If he did, some review procedure might be necessary, as discussed below.) The person in whose favour the power of attorney is executed is likely to be close to the patient. It is not impossible that he might be subconsciously influenced by improper considerations, for example, the prospect of release from the burden of caring for the patient at home. Persons who have an interest (financial or otherwise) in the patient's fate might be prevented from acting as witnesses, but it would be difficult to exclude them from the power of decision-making under a durable power of attorney, because an 'interested party' is the very person most patients would choose.

(d) *Procedure*
It is likely that the procedure for creating a durable power of attorney (see, for example, the Enduring Powers of Attorney Act 1985) will be more cumbersome than the procedure for executing a living will declaration. This is inevitable if the necessary safeguards are to be incorporated. A degree of formality will, however, be required in both cases.

(e) *Lack of suitable agent*
It may be that some people, for example, childless widows or widowers, would have difficulty in finding a trusted person to act. A living will would obviously be more advantageous in such a case, but this does not detract from the advantages of a

durable power of attorney for those who do have a trusted friend or relative. One candidate could be a solicitor, but it may be doubted that such a person would have sufficiently intimate knowledge of the patient. For those with limited access to professional legal advice and with no suitable agent, the relative simplicity of a living will may have greater appeal.

(f) *Resources*

The question of resources has already been discussed and should not be regarded as a relevant consideration in deciding whether to choose living wills or durable powers of attorney. In any case it is thought that there is little distinction between them in the resources that are likely to be saved.

The above survey indicates that each option has its own advantages and disadvantages, so that it would not desirable to recommend living will legislation to the exclusion of durable power of attorney legislation or vice versa. The remainder of this section deals with the question whether the two options should be separately available, or used in combination, or both.

The advantages of the combined document are twofold:

(i) any uncertainty resulting from the drafting of the living will declaration (see (a) above) can be resolved by allowing the chosen agent, as opposed to the doctor, to make the decision;

(ii) the statement of wishes contained in the living will declaration provides guidance to the agent (assuming that he is to be guided by the patient's previously expressed wishes, as discussed below).

There is, however, a fundamental problem. If it is recommended that a living will declaration should not be mandatory, i.e. should take the form of a *request* only, then it is difficult to see what scope there could be for a durable power of attorney. The notion of an agent who has no legal power is unacceptable. It would therefore be impossible to have a combined instrument, part of which was not legally enforceable (the living will) and part of which was (the durable power). Even if the durable power were to be a separate instrument instead of part of the living will instrument, the position would still be unsatisfactory. If the preferred view is that there should be no legal force in a living will, then it should not be possible to achieve legal enforceability via a different route. The conclusion is that a durable power of attorney, either alone or in combination with a living will, can only be recommended, indeed, only makes sense, if the living will is to be legally binding. It is a matter of balancing, on the one hand, the reasons why a living will should be directory rather than mandatory with, on the other hand, the advantages which a durable power has over a living will, which would be lost if the living will is not to be legally binding.

If, in view of the above, it is concluded that the living will should be legally binding, further problems remain, in particular where a combined instrument is not used. It is possible to imagine a person creating more than one living will, or more than one durable power of attorney. The likely solution is, by analogy with the law of wills, that the later document would revoke the earlier either expressly or to the extent of any inconsistency. (See, for example, the Californian Durable Power of Attorney for Health Care Act 1983, which provides that a valid durable power of attorney for health care revokes any prior durable power of attorney for health care.) If a person executed a living will *and* a power of attorney in separate instruments, legislation should clarify whether the later document should revoke the earlier (assuming the order of execution is known), or whether the power of attorney should be construed as designed for the implementation of the living will.

Terms of a durable power of attorney

(a) *Drafting*

As with a living will, the problem is whether the instrument creating the power of attorney should attempt to be specific as to the types of treatment which the agent is empowered to sanction or refuse. Minimum requirements are that the instrument, or at any rate the legislation, should make clear what is the 'triggering event' and what are the criteria for decision-making. These two aspects are discussed below. Of course, the wording of the instrument will vary according to whether the durable power is created in isolation or in combination with a living will declaration. Set out below as examples, are (1) extracts from a Model Act (drawn up by the Legal Advisors Committee of Concern for Dying) containing guidelines as to how to create a durable power of attorney with definitions of the important terms used, and (2) a combined document drawn up by the Society for the Right to Die.

APPENDIX
Right to Refuse Treatment Act

Section 1. Definitions

'Competent person' shall mean an individual who is able to understand and appreciate the nature and consequences of a decision to accept or refuse treatment.

'Declaration' shall mean a written statement executed according to the provisions of this Act which sets forth the declarant's intentions with respect to medical procedures, treatment or non-treatment, and may include the declarant's intentions concerning palliative care.

'Declarant' shall mean an individual who executes a declaration under the provisions of this Act.

'Health care provider' shall mean a person, facility or institution licensed or authorised to provide health care.

'Incompetent person' shall mean a person who is unable to understand and appreciate the nature and consequences of a decision to accept or refuse treatment.

'Medical procedure or treatment' shall mean any action taken by a physician or health care provider designed to diagnose, assess, or treat a disease, illness, or injury. These include, but are not limited to, surgery, drugs, transfusions, mechanical ventilation, dialysis, resuscitation, artificial feeding, and any other medical act designed for diagnosis, assessment or treatment.

'Palliative care' shall mean any measure taken by a physician or health care provider designed primarily to maintain the patient's comfort. These include, but are not limited to, sedatives and pain-killing drugs: non-artificial, oral feeding; suction; hydration; and hygienic care.

'Physician' shall mean any physician responsible for the declarant's care.

Section 5.

A declarant shall have the right to appoint in the declaration a person authorised to order the administration, withholding, or withdrawal of medical procedures and treatment in the event that the declarant become incompetent. A person so authorised shall have the power to enforce the provisions of the declaration and shall be bound to exercise the authority consistent with the declaration and the authorised person's best judgment as to the actual desires and preferences of the declarant. No palliative care measure may be withheld by an authorised person unless explicitly provided for in the declaration. Physicians and health care providers caring for incompetent declarants shall provide such authorised persons all medical information which would be available to the declarant if the declarant were competent.

(1) Extracts from a Model Act. Reprinted by permission of the Legal Advisors Committee of Concern for Dying, Boston.

Society for the Right to Die

250 West 57th Street/New York, NY 10107

Living Will Declaration

To My Family, Doctors, and All Those Concerned with My Care

INSTRUCTIONS
Consult this column for help and guidance.

I, _____, being of sound mind, make this statement as a directive to be followed if I become unable to participate in decisions regarding my medical care.

This declaration sets forth your directions regarding medical treatment.

If I should be in an incurable or irreversible mental or physical condition with no reasonable expectation of recovery, I direct my attending physician to withhold or withdraw treatment that merely prolongs my dying. I further direct that treatment be limited to measures to keep me comfortable and to relieve pain.

You have the right to refuse treatment you do not want, and you may request the care you do want.

These directions express my legal right to refuse treatment. Therefore I expect my family, doctors, and everyone concerned with my care to regard themselves as legally and morally bound to act in accord with my wishes, and in so doing to be free of any legal liability for having followed my directions.

You may list specific treatment you do __not__ want. For example:

Cardiac resuscitation
Mechanical respiration
Artificial feeding/fluids by tubes

Otherwise, your general statement, top right, will stand for your wishes.

I especially do not want: _____

_____

_____

_____

_____

_____

You may want to add instructions for care you __do__ want—for example, pain medication; or that you prefer to die at home if possible.

Other instructions/comments: _____

_____

_____

_____

Proxy Designation Clause: Should I become unable to communicate my instructions as stated above, I designate the following person to act in my behalf:

Name_____

Address_____

If you want, you can name someone to see that your wishes are carried out, but you do not have to do this.

If the person I have named above is unable to act in my behalf, I authorize the following person to do so:

Name_____

Address_____

Sign and date here in the presence of two adult witnesses, who should also sign.

Signed: _____ Date: _____

Witness: _____ Witness: _____

Keep the signed original with your personal papers at home. Give signed copies to doctors, family, and proxy. Review your Declaration from time to time; initial and date it to show it still expresses your intent.

- -

(2) A combined document. Reprinted by permission of the Society for the Right to Die, 250 West 57 Street, New York 10107.

The conclusion of the President's Commission Report was that 'by combining a proxy directive with specific instructions, an individual could control both the content and the process of decision-making about care in case of incapacity' (pp. 155–60). Although no specific form of document is included, the Model Act attempts to put this into effect by 'permitting the declarant both to define what interventions are refused, and to name an authorised individual to make decisions consistent with the declarant's desires as expressed in the declaration'. Thus Section 1 defines 'competent person', 'medical procedure or treatment' and 'palliative care', and then Section 5 gives the declarant the right to appoint a person to order the administration, withholding or withdrawing of the defined treatments. The trigger is incompetence, and the criterion is 'substituted judgment' (explained below). It seems that these provisions meet the minimum standards of certainty.

As far as the combined document is concerned, it will be seen that the 'trigger' is inability to participate in decisions regarding medical care, 'life-sustaining procedures' are defined, and that, by implication, the criterion is 'substituted judgment' (although this should preferably be expressly stated). The area of uncertainty, however, seems to lie in the second paragraph of the living will declaration ('I direct . . . meaningful quality of life').

Turning to the Californian statute on Durable Power of Attorney for Health Care 1983, the Act defines 'health care', the 'trigger' is the principal's inability to give informed consent in respect to the particular decision, and the criterion is 'substituted judgment' unless the desires of the principal are unknown, in which case it is 'best interests' (explained below). No particular form of wording is prescribed, except that printed forms sold for use by a person who does not have legal advice must contain a warning notice specified in the Act, and the Act specifies a form of wording which must (in substance) be adopted in the declaration of the witnesses or the notary public, as the case may be.

(b) *The 'triggering event'*

The basic question is whether the durable power of attorney should come into operation merely upon the supervening incompetence of the principal, or whether some further event should be required, for example terminal illness or some other kind of illness. The question of the triggering event has already been considered in relation to living wills (see page 52), and definitions of competence and incompetence were considered at length in Chapter 3. Therefore, these issues will not be examined in detail here. For present purposes, suffice it to say that the definitions adopted for durable powers of attorney should be the same as those which apply to living wills and to any code of practice dealing with the treatment of competent and incompetent persons.

(c) *The criterion for decision-making by the agent*

This is a matter of choosing between 'substituted judgment' and 'best interests'. The 'substituted judgment' criterion is where the agent's decision is based on the known wishes of the principal, i.e. the agent makes the decision which the principal would have made but for his incompetence. The 'best interest' test is different, as that requires a decision which, objectively, is deemed to be in the best interests of the principal, even if it is not the decision he would have made.

As far as the treatment of incompetents generally is concerned, it may be that 'best interests' is the preferable test because if a person has never been competent, it is a matter of speculation as to what he or she would have decided if competent. (See, for example, discussion of this point in the Canadian case of *Eve* [1986] considered in Chapter 3.) However, in the present case we are dealing with people who have been competent, and who are likely to have made their wishes known. For this reason the 'substituted judgment' test is to be preferred. This was the view of the President's Commission Report:

The Commission believes that, when possible, decision-making for incapacitated patients should be guided by the principle of substituted judgment, which promotes the underlying values of self-determination and well-being better than the best interests standard does. When a patient's likely decision is unknown, however, a surrogate decision-maker should use the best interests standard and choose a course that will promote the patient's well-being as it would probably be conceived by a reasonable person in the patient's circumstances. On certain points, of course, no consensus may exist about what most people would prefer, and surrogates retain discretion to choose among a range of acceptable choices (p. 136).

Substituted judgment is the standard applied in the Concern for Dying Model Act and in the Californian Durable Power of Attorney for Health Care Act 1983, which provides that the attorney has a duty to act 'consistent with the desires of the principal as expressed in the durable power of attorney or otherwise made known to the attorney in fact at any time or, if the principal's desires are unknown, to act in the best interests of the principal'.

When the durable power is combined with a living will declaration, the arguments for applying the substituted judgment test are even stronger. However one consequence of adopting this criterion might be that there would be no scope for taking non-medical matters into account (see page 62). Even if the best interests standards were adopted, it is unclear whether such matters could be considered in the absence of express statutory provision.

Practical and procedural matters

The practical and procedural matters already discussed on pages 56–60, in relation to living wills, apply equally or very similarly to durable powers of attorney. These will not be dealt with again. However, there are a number of additional matters which are relevant to durable powers of attorney alone.

(a) *Capacity of agent*

As with the principal, the agent should be a competent adult, the test for competence presumably being the same in each case. However in a recent judgment relating to the Enduring Powers of Attorney Act 1985, the test of competence applied to the principal was a low one, and lower than that required of the agent.[17] Another question is whether it should be possible to have *joint* agents in order to provide a further safeguard. In the Law Commission report on the Incapacitated Principal, the notion that joint attorneys should be *compulsory* was rejected.[18] The Enduring Powers of Attorney Act 1985 does, however, *permit* joint agents. It is suggested that this is too cumbersome and that only one should be appointed.

(b) *Witnesses*
Clearly the person in whose favour the power of attorney is executed should not be a witness. Reference has already been made (see pages 56–7, section (c)) to the difficulty that would arise if potential beneficiaries were to be excluded not merely from witnessing but from acting under the power of attorney.

(c) *Forms*
It has already been suggested that the durable power of attorney must be in writing, signed and witnessed. As discussed on page 69, section (a), it does not seem necessary that the document should be in prescribed form. Nor does it seem necessary that there should be a requirement of prior discussion with an informed official, though this would usually be desirable. However, there may be a case for requiring the document to contain explanatory information, for the protection of the principal, in the case where printed power of attorney forms are available to the public at large (see the 1983 Californian Act). It should be noted that the Enduring Powers of Attorney Act 1985 requires both a prescribed form and the incorporation of explanatory information.

(d) *Revocation*
The main issues have already been discussed on pages 58–9, section (h), and the following are additional points, relevant to durable powers of attorney.

The execution of a durable power should revoke any earlier power, and dissolution of marriage should revoke the appointment of the spouse as agent. This is analogous to the law of wills and is also found in the Californian Act of 1983.

In considering whether the principle should be entitled to revoke if he becomes incompetent, the President's Commission Report took the view that he should have power to override the agent as far as life-sustaining treatment is concerned. The Model Act (Section 6) permits revocation without specifying any requirement for continuing capacity.

The Californian Act of 1983 seems to achieve a compromise. On the one hand it provides that the principal can only revoke if he still has capacity (although there is a rebuttable presumption that he does). On the other hand, it further provides that the agent has no authority to consent to or refuse health care necessary to keep the principal alive if the principal objects. In such a case, the matter is governed by the law that would apply if there were no durable power of attorney. This seems to be the most satisfactory solution.

(e) *Limits on the agent's power*
The question arises whether certain matters should be excluded from the agent's sphere of authority. This could be done by limiting his role to 'life-sustaining procedures' (which must be defined), as with the combined living will and power of attorney form (above), or in some other way. There is much to be said for the provision in the Model Act that he cannot authorise the withholding of palliative care unless the instrument expressly so provides. It is unlikely however, that there is any justification here for excluding such matters as are excluded in the Californian Act of 1983, for example psychosurgery. The agent should not have any power to make decisions, including consent to abortion, if the principal is pregnant.

There must also be provision for allowing the doctor to give emergency treatment without consulting the agent. (See the Californian Act 1983.)

(f) *Delegation by the agent*
If the agent is temporarily or permanently unable or unwilling

to act (as to which, see also Disclaimer, below) the question arises as to whether he can delegate. The President's Commission Report (p. 151) suggests such a possibility. It is thought, however, that this is undesirable. The principal should be able to choose a 'reserve' (see the combined living will/power of attorney document discussed on pages 68–9) but if he does not, the position will be as if no durable power existed if the agent cannot or will not act.

(g) *Disclaimer by the agent*
It would seem impossible to provide that the agent is to be compelled to make a decision. When the time comes he may not wish to take the responsibility. The Californian Act 1983 does not seem to provide for this, but the Enduring Powers of Attorney Act 1985 allows disclaimer by permitting the agent to give notice to the principal while the latter is still competent, or, if he is not, by notice to the court. Disclaimer by notice to the competent principal seems unobjectionable, but a requirement of notice to the court in the present context seems too cumbersome. It is suggested that if the agent declines to act and no reserve has been designated by the principal, then the position will be as if no durable power existed.

(h) *Can the agent's decision be challenged?*
What happens if there is a suspicion of bad faith, or an apparently unreasonable interpretation of the principal's wishes? The President's Commission Report (pp. 152–3) suggests the possibility of an independent review, either 'intrainstitutional' or by way of court proceedings. Certainly the principal's interests must be safeguarded, but the notion of review by the court seems cumbersome. The statute could perhaps provide for review by a body such as the hospital ethics committee, on specified grounds, for example where the agent has not applied the correct criterion (see pages 70–1, section (c)) to his decision.

(i) *Medical records*
Should the agent be entitled to see the principal's records? He must have the necessary information in order to make a

decision, but, on the other hand, the principal's privacy must be respected. Taking the latter point into account, the President's Commission Report suggests that it may be advisable to limit the agent's access to information needed for the particular decision in question. This may not work, since the agent may not know what is relevant until he has looked at everything. The Californian Act 1983 provides that the agent has the same right as the principal to receive information, unless the right is limited in the instrument creating the power. The Model Act is on similar lines. It is thought that this is preferable to the suggestion of the President's Commission.

(j) *Notice to relatives*

The Enduring Powers of Attorney Act 1985 provides that the agent is obliged to notify various relatives when he applies to register the power (which he must do when he believes the principal is or is becoming incompetent). The relatives then have a chance to object on certain grounds, for example that the power is invalid, or the principal is not incompetent. This obviously provides an extra safeguard, but would probably be too cumbersome in the present context, especially if provision is made for a review procedure (see (h) above).

References

1. Gutheil, T. A., Bursztajn, H., and Brodsky, A. (1984). Malpractice prevention through the sharing of uncertainty. Informed consent and the therapeutic alliance. *New England Journal of Medicine*, 311: 49–51.
2. Gilmore, A. (1985). The nature of informed consent. *Canadian Medical Association Journal*, 132: 1198–203.
3. *In re Quinlan* 355 A 2d 647 [1976].
4. *In re Conroy* 486 A 2d 1209 [1985].
5. *Attorney General of British Columbia* v. *Astaforoff* [1984] 4 WWR 385.
6. *Re W (EEM)* [1971] ch. 123, 143 per Ungoed-Thomas J.
7. Stone, A. A. (1985). Law's influence on medicine and medical ethics. *New England Journal of Medicine*, 312: 309–12.
8. Parsons, A. (1985). Allocating health care resources: A moral dilemma. *Canadian Medical Association Journal*, 132: 466–9.
9. Stone, A. A. op. cit.
10. Weisbard, A. J. (1986). Defensive law. A new perspective on informed consent. *Archives of Internal Medicine*, 146: 860–61.

11. Redleaf, D. L., Schmitt, S. B., and Thompson, W. C. (1979). The California Natural Death Act: An empirical study of physicians' practices. *Stanford Law Review*, 31: 913–945.

12. Spencer, S. S. (1979). 'Code' or 'No Code': A non-legal opinion. *New England Journal of Medicine*, 300: 138–40.

13. Legal Advisors Committee of Concern for Dying (1983). The right to refuse treatment: A model act. *American Journal of Public Health*, 73: 918–21.

14. The President's Commission Report (1983). *Deciding to Forego Life-Sustaining Treatment*, p. 147. US Government Printing Office, Washington D.C.

15. The President's Commission Report, op. cit., p. 145.

16. The Legal Advisors Committee of Concern for Dying, op. cit.

17. Cf. *In re K: In re F*, on the Enduring Powers of Attorney Act 1985 [1988] 1 All ER 358.

18. Law Commission Report No. 122, para. 3.27. (1983). *The Incapacitated Principal*, Cmnd 8977. HMSO, London.

5 Conclusions

Introduction

During the discussion involved in the preparation of this report, it became apparent that although certain issues could be resolved and proposals made, it would, perhaps, be precipitate to attempt to offer a comprehensive set of recommendations. The absence of any previous experience of advance directives for health care in the UK calls for caution at the present stage in suggesting the precise steps which should be taken. The issues involved are sensitive and complex, and experience from abroad, although helpful, should not be regarded as directly applicable to this country. Furthermore the States of the USA which have most experience with advance directives are still developing and modifying their law and practice and evaluating their effects.

Thus, the purpose of this final chapter will not be to make a single set of recommendations supporting any one point of view. Rather the aim will be to demonstrate the range of options available and to summarise the principal arguments for and against each of them. This will allow a judgment to be made as to which course of action is likely to prove the most suitable in achieving the object which originally prompted our consideration of advance directives.

The options available

The range of options available (which are not all mutually exclusive) is as follows:

(1) to do nothing, on the basis that there is no demand or need for change;

(2) to advocate changes in medical practice, to ensure that it conforms with the ethical and legal framework outlined in Chapter 3;

(3) to introduce living wills on either a statutory or non-statutory basis, and to make their provisions either directory or mandatory;

(4) to introduce durable powers of attorney by statute, the basis of the agent's decision-making being either that of 'substituted judgment' or of 'best interests';

(5) to introduce by statute living wills combined with a durable power of attorney.

The advantages and disadvantages of these various options will now be considered.

The status quo

The main principle of autonomy which underlies proposals for advance directives concerns the importance of patients having the right to make decisions about their own health care. If this is accepted, present medical practice relating to incompetent patients cannot be considered satisfactory, firstly, because many doctors do not respect the autonomy of their patients but act on what they, the doctors, consider to be their patients' best interests, and secondly because for incompetent patients there is normally no mechanism by which their wishes concerning their health care can be known. In theory a patient can convey his wishes to his general practitioner, who will take note of them should he become incompetent, but there is no evidence that this is a common practice.

Surveys have shown that most people do not think that doctors should always provide every available treatment to keep them alive (see Chapters 1 and 2). This does not, however, imply that there is necessarily a demand for change, as there is no good evidence about whether patients wish the final decision to be their own or be left to the doctors. Hence the likely demand for advance directives in the UK is uncertain. It could be argued, though, that even if only a small number of people wished to make use of advance directives, it should be possible to do so, on the principle that patient autonomy finds its most obvious expression in the exercise of choice.

What is certain is that there is a considerable variation in practice among doctors. Some doctors respect the autonomy of their patients whilst others act paternalistically, so that many patients must inevitably be dissatisfied with the doctor caring for them. It must be concluded that this situation warrants improvement.

Improving medical practice

The general improvement of services for the patients being considered does not in itself ensure that the interests of individual patients will necessarily be respected. This is particularly so when their wishes are unknown. In such cases doctors can only do what they consider to be in the patient's best interests. But, as we have seen, if this duty on the part of doctors is properly analysed and understood, it would enable doctors to accept that there are instances where both ethically and legally it is already good practice to forego further medical treatment. As a consequence, practice would change in a manner of which most people would approve. Resort to the tenets of good medical practice would not, of course, entirely obviate the need for advance directives. However, it might provide that degree of reassurance which many people seek and thereby limit the demand for advance directives. Such a change in practice is, therefore, best regarded as setting the context in which any move is made to introduce advance directives and complementary to it.

Although improvements in medical practice may remove some of the anxieties which reflect themselves in the call for advance directives, it is as well to notice that there is an objective element in the judgment of what is good medical practice. It does not necessarily consist of doing what each particular patient may demand. There is a limit to resources and a doctor has a duty to others. Thus, there is a limit to the treatment that a patient may demand. For example, not every patient may demand dialysis for renal failure and there must be a limit to the amount of very costly therapy a patient may demand for advanced cancer. Equally, a person who has written a living will or appointed an agent in respect of a durable power of attorney cannot demand that *everything* which could be done, must be done. The limits on care which are part of the concept of good medical practice must be regarded as the same as they would be for a competent patient. Advance directives must not be thought to confer privileges not otherwise available to patients, nor to impose on doctors obligations beyond those subsumed in good medical practice. Nor are they intended, and should not be understood, to be a means of commanding additional resources.

Living wills

The practical effect of legislation on living wills in the various states of the USA has not been widely evaluated, particularly as regards its influence on doctors' decision-making. In an early study of the California Natural Death Act, in a survey of 275 physicians, two-thirds said that the Act had made a difference to their clinical decisions about those patients who had signed a living will. However, there were considerable problems in the way that decision-making was influenced, so that benefits to patients were limited.[1] Part of the problem is that if living wills only provide for general directions they lack sufficient content to be of use in guiding the doctor, whereas if they contain specific instructions they may fail to provide for the precise event which subsequently occurs. This can be partly overcome by providing two sections for directions on the declaration forms, the first containing a general statement of the patient's wishes, and the second, which would be optional, containing more detailed directions. A standard form would meet these demands and ensure maximum effectiveness in drafting and is, therefore, to be recommended. Even with these provisions, however, the degree of influence on a doctor's decision-making will inevitably be less than optimal, and this is perhaps the most serious disadvantage of living wills.

There has been an additional and important effect of the legislation though, which may be termed cultural. Its effect has been general in making people more aware of the issues involved, and specific through the public education programmes which have been developed to accompany the legislation.

If living wills were to be recommended for use in the UK the question arises as to the basis on which they would be introduced. Should they be informal documents, which are merely advisory or exhortatory (i.e. without imposing any legal obligation on the doctor to follow the directions contained in them), or should they be introduced by statute, whether as advisory or mandatory documents? The advantages of the informal approach are:

(1) that it can be implemented immediately with a minimum of formal procedures;
(2) that it would allow for the ground to be tested, both in terms of public demand and of acceptability both to the public and doctors;
(3) that it would be more likely to be welcomed by doctors and professional medical organisations, than would legislation.

The disadvantages are:

(1) that it would have no force in law;
(2) that, as a consequence, it would not ensure that the doctor would follow the patient's directions and, being incompetent, the patient would have no means of challenging the doctor;
(3) that it could not provide for any directions which might go beyond that which is at present lawful;
(4) that the option of combining a living will with a durable power of attorney would be excluded, since, as has been seen, legislation is necessary to extend durable powers of attorney to decisions about treatment.

Durable powers of attorney

Durable powers of attorney, in the context of medical treatment, must be introduced by statute if the agent's authority is formally to be established and his directions become mandatory. This latter requirement is essential, since any other arrangement could lead to unresolvable disputes between the agent, relatives or other interested parties and the doctor. As discussed in Chapter 4, the criterion to be followed by the agent in his decision-making should be that of 'substituted judgment', rather than by reference to the patient's 'best interests'. In other words, the agent should attempt to be a sympathetic interpreter of the patient's wishes, rather than an objective judge of what would be in the patient's best interests. Equally, the agent should not act as an Ombudsman, arbitrating between the views of all the interested parties.

The principal advantage of durable powers of attorney over living wills is that it allows for the use of substituted judgment based on the circumstances which have arisen rather than being tied to the particular words of the living will, which may not entirely meet the situation at hand. Consequently, durable powers of attorney are likely to be more faithful in reflecting the patient's true wish and so respectful of patient autonomy. Their main disadvantage, on the other hand, is that a more complicated procedure is required so that they may appeal to fewer people than a living will. Also some people will not know a suitable person willing to act as their agent.

Living wills combined with durable powers of attorney

The accumulated experience in the USA suggests that if advance directives are introduced by statute, the most satisfactory approach is to combine living wills with durable powers of attorney, as the advantages of each then become complementary. The legislation involved would require that the directives were mandatory, as with the durable power of attorney alone. The main advantage of the combined document is that it allows the directions of the living will to be general, setting the context within which the agent named in the durable power of attorney will be guided as to how best to make detailed decisions in relation to the specific circumstances which arise in the particular case.

Protecting and promoting care

Throughout this report reference has been made to the importance of ensuring that those incompetent groups of patients for whose benefit advance directives would be introduced also receive a good standard of medical care. Access to such care is the first prerequisite. Medical care for the elderly and handicapped has come to be regarded as part of the 'Cinderella' services of the Health Service.

Improving the general level and quality of medical care is not in itself an alternative to the introduction of advance directives, but it is complementary to it, as well as being desirable in its own right. If the importance of improving services is not made clear there are a number of possible dangers in the way of getting advance directives accepted or of bringing them into disrepute. Firstly, people may be, or may feel, pressured into completing advance directives to enable resources to be saved. Secondly, some people may feel that to complete advance directives is one way of opting out of being potential recipients of services that they know or feel to be poor, and do not expect will be improved. Thirdly, if advance directives are introduced and become widely accepted, they could be used as a reason for reducing the level and standard of services to the patient groups involved.

Conversely, if services were improved, it might well be the case that the need or demand for advance directives would be reduced. The situation is analogous with that of terminal care and the apparent desire for euthanasia. Once the hospice movement and the concept and practice of treating for dying with high quality care had been generally introduced, the demand for solutions such as euthanasia may have been considerably lessened.

As the patients being considered generally suffer from the provision of poor services, it would be cynical to seek to introduce advance directives, without recognising at the same time the need for improvement of services. Indeed, a further step would be to consider legislation and other action to protect and promote the rights of incompetent patients.

As this report is not centrally concerned with the *general* care of incompetent patients, this proposal will not be considered in detail. However, we endorse the general recommendations put forward by Age Concern in its document *The Law and Vulnerable Elderly People*.[2] It recommends that local authorities be empowered to make specific provisions for vulnerable elderly people in the community. Furthermore, we draw attention to the legislation relating specifically to the partially and wholly incompetent which has recently been enacted in New Zealand, The Protection of Personal and Property Rights Act 1986. It empowers Family Courts to make specific orders in relation to the partially competent, and to appoint welfare guardians for the wholly incompetent. The courts could make orders about care or treatment which the person would not be able to demand or alternatively be unable to obtain despite being in need of it. As with the proposals of Age Concern, such legislation can only be successful if appropriate resources are made available, and this would apply to any similar recommendation.

The way forward

The main purpose of this report has been to set out the relevant medical, ethical and legal issues and to determine the terms of reference in considering advance directives as they relate to the United Kingdom. Certain specific matters have been resolved and unequivocal recommendations can be made. Firstly, whatever proposals are adopted they should be accompanied by general improvements in medical treatment and care for those conditions described, as outlined in Chapter 2. Secondly, there is a need to promote patient autonomy by the introduction of more specific measures involving advance directives, because for those who are permanently incompetent there is no other means by which this can be achieved. The decision whether to advocate that this should be by statutory or non-statutory means is more problematic. There are advantages and disadvantages to each, as previously described. If a non-statutory route is followed this must necessarily involve a living will on its own, and it would be preferable that a standardised form was introduced at a national level, with support from the government, the health care professions and the public. This would enable guidelines to be laid down about its use, so that the procedures involved in both writing and implementing living wills would become an established and well-recognised part of health care provision. If a statutory route is adopted, the weight of evidence from the USA supports a combined living will and durable power of attorney, the provisions of which are made mandatory.

We are only beginning the process of considering these issues in Britain and therefore think that the decision to follow a statutory or non-statutory route should only be made after a period of public and political debate. Accordingly, no firm recommendation will be made as to which should be adopted.

Conclusion

We have demonstrated that the changing pattern of modern medical practice in relation to those who become permanently incompetent and therefore incapable of making decisions about their own health care raises ethical and legal issues which require to be addressed in the interests of both patients and their doctors. We believe that these should be analysed in relation to the principle of respect for patient autonomy. After considering the complex issues involved, we have presented a number of proposals which would improve the quality of doctors' decision-making for these patients, especially as regards the withdrawing or withholding of life-saving or life-sustaining treatment.

It is our submission that these analyses and proposals warrant serious and critical deliberation and it is in that spirit that we recommend them.

References

1. Redleaf, D. L., Schmitt, S. B. and Thompson, W. C. (1979). The California Natural Death Act: An empirical study of physicians' practices, *Stanford Law Review*, 31: 913–45.
2. Age Concern (1986). *The Law and Vulnerable Elderly People*. Age Concern England, Surrey.

Recommendations

(1) Improvements should be made in medical treatment and care for all those who are terminally ill, seriously or permanently ill or disabled, and who have severe dementia. Two elements are involved: Firstly, the general protection and promotion of services for these groups of patients and, secondly, improvements in the individual care and management of patients.

(2) Advance directives for health care should be made available either on a statutory or a non-statutory basis. Extensive debate should be arranged amongst the public, the health care professions and politicians before any decision is taken to introduce advance directives nationally.

(3) A research programme should be launched to investigate:
  (a) the present state of medical practice in relation to the conditions being considered, with special regard to those who are permanently incompetent;
  (b) people's knowledge of the medical conditions under consideration, and their perception of the quality of their life should they develop these conditions and become permanently incompetent.

(4) An education and monitoring programme should be developed to accompany the introduction of advance directives, in order to inform the public about their use and determine their effectiveness in actualising the wishes which people express.

Appendix: Illustrative Cases

The following cases are illustrative of situations where an advance directive would have been of value in deciding the outcome:

Case 1: Terminal care

A 48-year-old woman developed a type of cancer which was treated initially by surgery and radiotherapy with an apparently good result. However, the disease recurred six months later and was treated by a course of chemotherapy near the end of which the patient suffered a stroke which paralysed one side of her body. About four months later, with no recovery of the paralysis and with further evidence of recurrence of the cancer, pneumonia developed. The doctors considered that the pneumonia should be treated, but the patient was no longer competent to make a meaningful decision. They consulted the patient's husband, who reasoned that the quality of his wife's previously very active life had now become so poor that, if capable, she would have refused treatment. No further treatment was given, and the patient died six days later.

Case 2: Serious and permanent disability

A retired judge suffered a severe stroke and was admitted to a general medical unit where he was in a coma for 48 hours. He regained consciousness, and when he opened his eyes his wife and sons were overjoyed. However, he made very little progress, and although he could understand simple words he could not speak. He was fed, lifted and washed, but was doubly incontinent. His wife devotedly helped with his care on the ward, and he was wheeled around and developed a mild interest in his surroundings. He gradually realised that he would be unable to return home, and all his interest failed. After two months he began to cry and wail constantly. He then stopped eating, refusing all nourishment by turning his head away and clamping his teeth. He became dehydrated and lost weight, and although he was unable to make his wishes known his relatives felt he was voluntarily 'giving up' and wanted to die. They wanted to respect his wishes and asked if his distress could be eased with drugs if he was literally starving.

A consultant psychiatrist was called and diagnosed profound depression, possibly amenable to treatment and said that a feeding tube should be passed into the stomach for the administration of food and antidepressant drugs. The family did not want to have their father tube fed.

The family were counselled and overruled, and amid great hostility on their part, a tube was passed. The patient survived and he was transferred to a rehabilitation unit where after a further two months he could sit upright in a wheelchair, was continent of faeces and could help his wife to transfer him. Six months after the stroke, the patient went home but he remained very disabled, and continued to be unable to communicate.

Case 3: Dementia

A 76-year-old retired school teacher developed progressive features of dementia, and after two years his wife, by now aged 79 and suffering a heart condition, was no longer able to cope with his serious physical and mental deterioration which included double incontinence.

He was admitted for assessment to a geriatric unit. A few weeks after admission, when the diagnosis of dementia had been confirmed, the man developed a high temperature and increasing drowsiness. Pneumonia was diagnosed and the doctors recommended treatment with an antibiotic. The man's wife and daughter disagreed and prevailed upon the doctors not to treat the pneumonia although the patient had never expressed any views about this sort of situation. The doctors only agreed because both the wife and daughter were formerly nurses, whose opinion they therefore respected. Thirty-six hours later the man died, in the words of his wife, 'peacefully and beautifully cared for'.

Index